CANCER ETIOLOGY, DIAGNOSIS AND TREATMENTS

QUANTUM BIOLOGY

METHODS TO CONVERT MALIGNANT CANCEROUS CELLS TO CELLS WITH REDUCED CpG METHYLATION THAT ARE ACCESSIBLE TO CANCER CELL-EATING SYSTEMS

CANCER ETIOLOGY, DIAGNOSIS AND TREATMENTS

Additional books and e-books in this series can be found on Nova's website under the Series tab.

CANCER ETIOLOGY, DIAGNOSIS AND TREATMENTS

QUANTUM BIOLOGY

METHODS TO CONVERT MALIGNANT CANCEROUS CELLS TO CELLS WITH REDUCED CpG METHYLATION THAT ARE ACCESSIBLE TO CANCER CELL-EATING SYSTEMS

KOHJI HASUNUMA PHD
GRADUATE SCHOOL OF INTEGRATED SCIENCE
YOKOHAMA CITY UNIVERSITY
YOKOHAMA, JAPAN

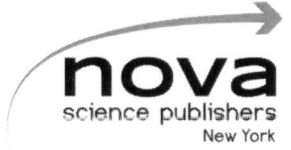

Copyright © 2019 by Nova Science Publishers, Inc.

All rights reserved. No part of this book may be reproduced, stored in a retrieval system or transmitted in any form or by any means: electronic, electrostatic, magnetic, tape, mechanical photocopying, recording or otherwise without the written permission of the Publisher.

We have partnered with Copyright Clearance Center to make it easy for you to obtain permissions to reuse content from this publication. Simply navigate to this publication's page on Nova's website and locate the "Get Permission" button below the title description. This button is linked directly to the title's permission page on copyright.com. Alternatively, you can visit copyright.com and search by title, ISBN, or ISSN.

For further questions about using the service on copyright.com, please contact:
Copyright Clearance Center
Phone: +1-(978) 750-8400　　　　Fax: +1-(978) 750-4470　　　　E-mail: info@copyright.com.

NOTICE TO THE READER

The Publisher has taken reasonable care in the preparation of this book, but makes no expressed or implied warranty of any kind and assumes no responsibility for any errors or omissions. No liability is assumed for incidental or consequential damages in connection with or arising out of information contained in this book. The Publisher shall not be liable for any special, consequential, or exemplary damages resulting, in whole or in part, from the readers' use of, or reliance upon, this material. Any parts of this book based on government reports are so indicated and copyright is claimed for those parts to the extent applicable to compilations of such works.

Independent verification should be sought for any data, advice or recommendations contained in this book. In addition, no responsibility is assumed by the Publisher for any injury and/or damage to persons or property arising from any methods, products, instructions, ideas or otherwise contained in this publication.

This publication is designed to provide accurate and authoritative information with regard to the subject matter covered herein. It is sold with the clear understanding that the Publisher is not engaged in rendering legal or any other professional services. If legal or any other expert assistance is required, the services of a competent person should be sought. FROM A DECLARATION OF PARTICIPANTS JOINTLY ADOPTED BY A COMMITTEE OF THE AMERICAN BAR ASSOCIATION AND A COMMITTEE OF PUBLISHERS.

Additional color graphics may be available in the e-book version of this book.

Library of Congress Cataloging-in-Publication Data

ISBN: 978-1-53614-775-9
Library of Congress Control Number: 2018965005

Published by Nova Science Publishers, Inc. † New York

*This book is dedicated to my research friend,
the late Doctor Mamoru Mimuro, who devoted his research career to
the analysis of photosynthesis. In response to my question, "How
should we address the problem of light from a molecular biological
perspective?" he answered to me, "We cannot answer this by
addressing the problem of light in the context of molecular biology."
This answer encouraged me to address problems in biology from
various perspectives, including that of "quantum biology."*

CONTENTS

Preface		ix
Introduction		xiii
Acknowledgements		xvii
Chapter 1	Functions of the Nucleoside Diphosphate Kinase (NDPK-1), the Superoxide Dismutase, and the Catalase in *Neurospora crassa*	1
Chapter 2	Functional Analyses of the Human (*Homo sapiens*) Nucleoside Diphosphate Kinase (NDPK), the Superoxide Dismutase, and the Catalase	35
Concluding Remarks		79
About the Author		81
Index		83

PREFACE

From the context of a molecular biological perspective, several biological phenomena have remained unresolved. I would like to address a part of such fundamental phenomena. In plants, the concentration of unsaturated fatty acids constituting membrane systems is unusually high such as (i.e., 80%). There is no explanation from a molecular biological perspective for this phenomenon. However, we should realize that singlet oxygen ($^1O_2$) is generated via an excitation through photo-activated chlorophyll (triplet chlorophyll) in sunlight and by the functional processes of H_2O photolysis to generate triplet oxygen ($^3O_2$).

$$2H_2O \rightarrow 4H^+ + 4e^- + {}^3O_2$$

Triplet oxygen ($^3O_2$) will accept enough energy from triplet-chlorophyll to provide energy to two fluctuating energy states of $^1O_2$, namely, $^1\Delta g$ and $^1\Sigma g^+$, and emitted in the range of 200 - 500 μm. The half-life of $^1O_2$ is 0.5 - 4 μs. The energy of $^1O_2$ is alleviated by unsaturated fatty acids present in various membrane systems, including plasma membranes, chloroplast thylakoids, the mitochondrial envelope membrane, and the nuclear membrane. The terminal end of unsaturated fatty acids with double bonding can react at the double bonded with $^1O_2$

to form malondialdehyde (MDA). However, there is no such description of this process in "Molecular Biology" (Hasunuma 2017).

In humans (*Homo sapiens*), the methylation of CpG islands in cancerous cells is so high that the sensing capacity of the genes with CpG islands (placed roughly 30 kbp upstream of the genes to sense ambient circumstantial changes of the circumstance responding genes with CpG islands), in their microenvironment would be hindered. Rather, housekeeping genes function independently, sensing various types of information from neighboring cells, and supporting the proliferation of cells behaving as cancerous cells, and the cells become those which are in a malignant and develop a metastatic state. The CpG island-controlled genes (45,000 in the human haploid genome) and CpG island-independent genes (35,000 in the human haploid genome) co-regulate to each other in the normal cell systems (Antequera and Bird 1993).

FAD (flavin adenine dinucleotide), FMN (flavin mononucleotide), riboflavin, and derivatives of heme groups are well known as the photosensitizers. They emit $^1O_2$ with reactive oxygen species (ROS), *in vivo*. In sunlight, as described above, photosensitizers will function as the generators of $^1O_2$ and ROS. From a clinical perspective, during the daytime, there is a plentiful supply of $^1O_2$ and ROS from the sunlight, and which inevitably contributes to the circadian rhythms of second messengers originating from the mutual regulation of second messengers (Hasunuma 1991, Hasunuma et al. 2005, Yoshida et al. 2006, Yoshida et al. 2011). In the latter two papers, there was no such description in terms of the "molecular biology." The repeated evolution of $^1O_2$, and ROS, and further additional second messengers might be closely associated with the development of an embryo. Nucleoside diphosphate kinase (NDPK), which is demonstrated to be involved in the process of detoxifying $^1O_2$, influences the circadian rhythm for conidiation in *Neurospora crassa*. Further, the thorax formation process in *Drosophila melanogaster* as presenting with an abnormal wing disc formation (*AWD*) includes nucleoside diphosphate kinase (NDPK), which is demonstrated to be a component of detoxification in the process of detoxifying $^1O_2$.

The tubulin structures, extending from the plasma membrane to two centrosomes located along the sides of the nucleus, which have like a structure similar to that of the sunrays radiating strong light, with stripes of light irradiation, and are designated as asters. In dark conditions, the protein complex of NDPK-1/catalase is located at the plasma membrane. However, upon light illumination, the NDPK-1/catalase protein complex moves along the aster, forming the tubulin structures towards the cytosol. As a result, the nucleus is protected from $^1O_2$ by the wall composed of the NDPK-1/catalase complex (Roymans et al. 2000). The CpG islands in the nucleus can be protected from methylation induced by the $^1O_2$ molecules generated in the neighboring cells harboring photosensitizers, such as FAD, FMN, riboflavin, and derivatives of porphyrin, including such as the open tetrapyrrole and heme groups.

From these phenomena, I have deduced that plants ultimately require sunlight and this requirement is almost perfectly addressed by introducing the fundamental considerations of "quantum physics in biology." The requirement of light illumination in animal science is also completely dependent on the light illumination, although photosynthesis does not occur in "animals."

INTRODUCTION

Singlet oxygen ($^1O_2$) generated via photosensitizers from triplet oxygen ($^3O_2$) is emitted in a range of 200 – 500 μm.

The summary of the report by (Hasunuma 2017) is as follows: "Light energy transduction causes the excitation of the energy state of triplet oxygen ($^3O_2$), generated by photolysis of H_2O to singlet oxygen ($^1O_2$) via the photosensitizers, FAD, FMN, riboflavin, and open tetrapyrrole (a kind of heme group and also porphyrin), and giving the resultant emissions of $^1O_2$ in the range of 200 – 500 μm." The $^1O_2$ entering into the neighboring cells is captured by cytosolic or plasma membrane-bound catalase, which forms protein complexes with nucleoside diphosphate kinase (NDPK). Catalase has the ability to bind $^1O_2$ and NADPH, and the NDPK has the ability to interact with catalase and bind NADH. The bound NADH can transfer electrons to the catalase bound to $^1O_2$, to release super oxide (O_2^-). Singlet oxygen entering through the plasma membrane and the monolayer of the endoplasmic reticulum can react with the unsaturated fatty acids in the membranes and form compounds, such as malondialdehyde, which destroys the membrane integrity and permits the release of Ca^{2+}. The increase in [Ca^{2+}] cyt initiates successive reactions that result in defining the circadian rhythm. These reaction sequences would alleviate the damages caused by strong sunlight, resulting in high yielding. In contrast, where as shown in a high-yielding mutant *R3-1* in *Pisum,* which had point mutations in the transit peptide and in the enzyme, NDPK-2 (I12L, E205K), it had elevated autophosphorylation and enzyme activities. High-yielding mutants, therefore, had an enhanced capacity to reduce the damage caused by strong sunlight.

The triplet oxygen ($^3O_2$) generated by photolysis of water is excited by triplet chlorophylls, which emits $^1O_2$ in the range of 200 – 500 μm. The $^1O_2$ will modify deoxy-guanosine to 8-hydroxy-deoxy-guanosine, which stimulates the modification of neighboring deoxy-cytosines to be modified to 5-methyl-deoxy-cytosines in the presence of DNA methyltransferase, with S-adenosyl-methyonine being used as a methyl donor. The regulation of the methylation of CpG islands, which regulates the genetic expression of DNA in the neighboring cells, will initiate differentiation in these cells. Singlet oxygen is, not only generated by photosensitizers, including FAD, FMN, riboflavin, and heme groups such as open tetrapyrrole, but also by the excitation reaction of the photolysis of H_2O-generated triplet oxygen ($^3O_2$) to singlet oxygen ($^1O_2$), and it contributes to the programming of differentiation in plant cells, and the initiation of structural differentiation.

Possible therapeutic administration of anti-oxidation reagents would reduce the rate of flux of $^1O_2$.

(a) Human and mouse cancerous diseases are under the control of the biological rhythm, achieved using major factors of reactive oxygen species (ROS), including $^1O_2$.

Light energy transduction, resulting in a circadian rhythm, with the oscillation of ROS (including $^1O_2$) in *Neurospora crassa,* was demonstrated by Yoshida et al. (2010). These conserved circadian rhythms are possibly operating in humans and mice.

(b) Photoreceptors, including FAD, FMN, riboflavin, and derivatives of porphyrin, such as open tetrapyrrol and also heme-groups.

These photoreceptors can function as photosensitizers and will emit ROS, including $^1O_2$, in humans and mice exposed to sunlight.

(c) Singlet oxygen ($^1O_2$) induced DNA methylation in cancerous cells.

In cancerous cells, most of the CpG islands located upstream of circumstance responsive genes (45,000 in human haploid genome) are heavily methylated, and most of these genes are down regulated or in some cases up regulated, with no further changes in gene regulation. Therefore, only house-keeping genes with no CpG island those that contribute to cell proliferation (35,000 in human haploid genome) would be functioning, and these cells will continue to proliferate as un-controlled cancerous cells (Antequera and Bird 1993). Singlet oxygen ($^1O_2$) directly reacts with deoxy-G in CpG islands and forms 8-hydroxy-deoxy-guanosine, which will stimulates the methylation of deoxy-C to form 5-methyl-deoxy-cytosine by DNA-methyltransferase, using S-adenosyl-methionine as the methyl donor (Cerda and Weitzman 1997, Wachsman 1997).

(d) Singlet oxygen ($^1O_2$) detoxification and de-methylation of DNA by long noncoding RNA.

Hydroxyl methylation and noncoding RNA can stimulate the de-methylation of DNA, and these factors can function as cancer curing factors of cancerous cells. The hyper-methylation of CpG islands is not fixed, but rather, it is reversed, resulting in de-methylated CpG islands (Mercer et al. 2009).

(e) Proposed reagents related for the detoxification of singlet oxygen ($^1O_2$).

Administration of NDPK proteins, such as Nm23-H1, Nm23-H2, catalase proteins, and Cu, Zn, superoxide dismutase should be administered to cancerous cell cultures, and this should be followed by the administration of unsaturated fatty acids, NADH, and NADPH, the $^1O_2$ scavengers, tocopherol (vitamin E), and β-carotene, and vitamin C should be administered for the detoxification of $^1O_2$. Vitamin C will support the detoxification of ROS, such as OH· group, in cancerous cells, preventing the further metastasis of malignant cancerous cells.

The detoxification of $^1O_2$ permits the de-methylation of the CpG islands. The weakened cancerous cells, which will respond to the changes in the environment, may be eaten by cancer cell-eating systems, such as B-cells and T-cells.

The actual experiments would be carried out with human and mouse cancerous cell cultures, adding the corresponding human and mouse NDPKs, catalase proteins, Cu, Zn superoxide dismutase, unsaturated fatty acids, co-factors NADH and NADPH, and the $^1O_2$ scavengers, tocopherol (vitamin E) and β-carotene, would be added, along with and the detoxification assisting factor, vitamin C.

ACKNOWLEDGEMENTS

Sincere gratitude is extended to Winslow R. Briggs and to Noboru Takasugi for their continuous encouragements, and to Tatsuo Ishikawa for initiating this work.

Sincere gratitude is extended to the following individuals:

Co-workers:
Yusuke Yoshida: PhD, Yokohama City University, Japan;
Emdadul Haque: PhD, Yokohama City University, Japan.

Reviewed by:
Mitsuhiro Yamada: PhD, The University of Tokyo, Japan;
Hideo Mohri: PhD, The University of Tokyo, Japan.

Chapter 1

FUNCTIONS OF THE NUCLEOSIDE DIPHOSPHATE KINASE (NDPK-1), THE SUPEROXIDE DISMUTASE, AND THE CATALASE IN *NEUROSPORA CRASSA*

1.1. FUNCTIONS OF THE NUCLEOSIDE DIPHOSPHATE KINASE (NDPK) AND THE CATALASE IN *NEUROSPORA CRASSA*

The genes for NDPK-1 and the mutant protein NDPK-1^{P72H} were named *ndpk-1* and *ndpk-1^{P72H}*, respectively. The functions of these proteins are described in the following section.

An *in vitro* assay system of the protein developed by Oda and Hasunuma (1994, 1997) revealed that the phosphorylation of a 15-kDa protein (NDPK-1) caused an increase in the phosphorylation because in response to exposure to blue light illumination for 1 s. The reaction was performed in a mixture containing 4 ×10^{-9} M of carrier-free [γ-^{32}P]ATP on ice. After mixing the reaction mixture with the crude membrane fraction of mycelia, the reaction was carried out on ice. After 5 s with or without illuminating to the reaction mixture, sodium dodecyl sulfate (SDS) sample buffer was added to stop the reaction, which was then subjected to a 5-20% sucrose gradient SDS-poly acrylamide gel electrophoresis (PAGE). The results are schematically presented in Figure 1.1.1.

The genes for encoding catalase, namely, *cat-1*, *cat-2*, *cat-3*, and *cat-4*, and their corresponding enzyme proteins, Cat-1, Cat-2, Cat-3, and Cat-4 were identified in *N. crassa*. The light-induced interactions between Cat-1, Cat-2, and Cat-3 with NDPK-1 or with NDPK-1^{P72H}, while responding to light-induced phenomena, were also described. As it was difficult to demonstrate the presence of Cat-4, the description for it has not been included in the review.

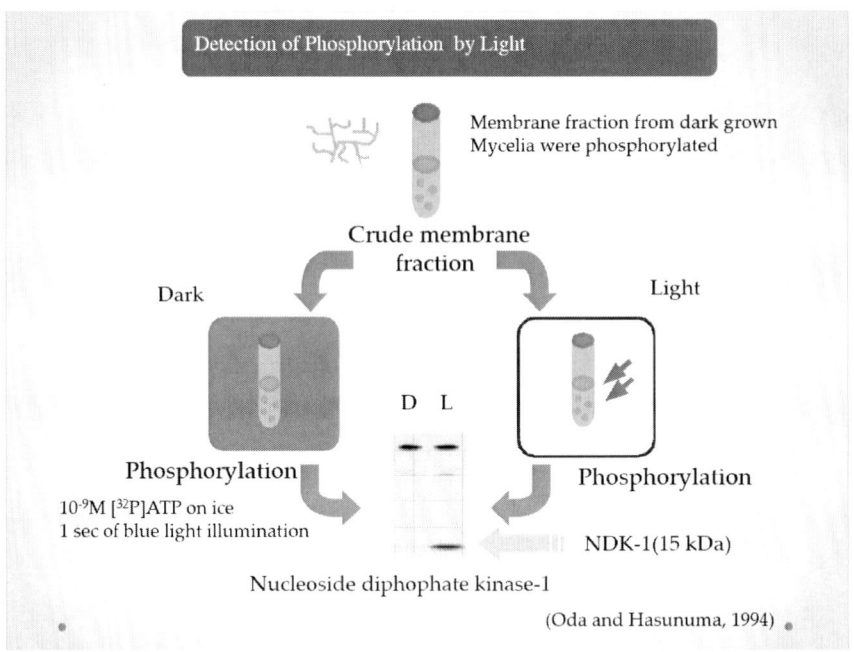

Figure 1.1.1. Schematic representation of the detection of light energy transduction in *N. crassa*.

Using a yeast two-hybrid method, the effective interactions between the C-terminal half of AtNDPK1 with AtCAT1, AtCAT2 and AtCAT3 were detected in *Arabidopsis thaliana* (Fukamatsu et al. 2003).

Catalase is a heme-protein and constitutes homo-tetramers. Each monomer can bind singlet oxygen ($^1O_2$), which can be differentiated by performing the detection using native PAGE, based on the faster movement of the protein band; the more with acidification of proteins by the binding of $^1O_2$, the faster the mobilization of the protein in native PAGE. Catalase proteins with and without $^1O_2$ can be detected by soaking the native gel into a specific reagent, and H_2O_2 catalyzing activity can also be detected using this system (Yoshida et al. 2006).

1.2. DIFFERENTIATION OF PROTOPERITHECIA, OF AERIAL HYPHA TO MACROCONIDIA, AND OF THICK MYCELIA TO MACROCONIDIA IN *N. CRASSA*

Protoperithecia are the female sexual organs in *N. crassa*, which are formed independently of the "A" or "a" mating type in the medium containing low concentrations of nitrogen, such as, the Westergaard medium. Microconidia, macroconidia, and mycelia are the male organs.

Blue or white light-stimulated processes are summarized as follows.

(1) Carotenoid formation in the mycelia and in the aerial hyphae is enhanced (Yoshida and Hasunuma 2004).
(2) Aerial hyphae and macroconidial formation from thick mycelia are stimulated by blue light (Lee et al. 2006).
(3) The formation of the female organ, protoperithecium, is stimulated by blue light (Lee et al. 2006).

(4) Standing development of perithecia from protoperithecia is stimulated by blue or white light presented laterally from the side (Ogura et al. 2001).
(5) Bending of the perithecial beak toward light is stimulated by blue or white light (Ogura et al. 2001).
(6) The phase shift of the circadian rhythm of conidiation is stimulated by blue or white light (Yoshida et al. 2008).
(7) The conidiation rhythm of the *band* is suppressed (singularity response) by light pulse (Huang et al. 2006).
(8) Carotenoid synthesis under blue light is stimulated by the presence of oxygen under blue light. However, the stimulation of carotenoid synthesis was not observed when air was replaced with N_2 gas (Iigusa et al. 2005).
(9) The circadian rhythm for conidiation is dependent on riboflavin, as is evident by the presence of *band, rib-1* and *band, rib-2* (Frits et al. 1989).

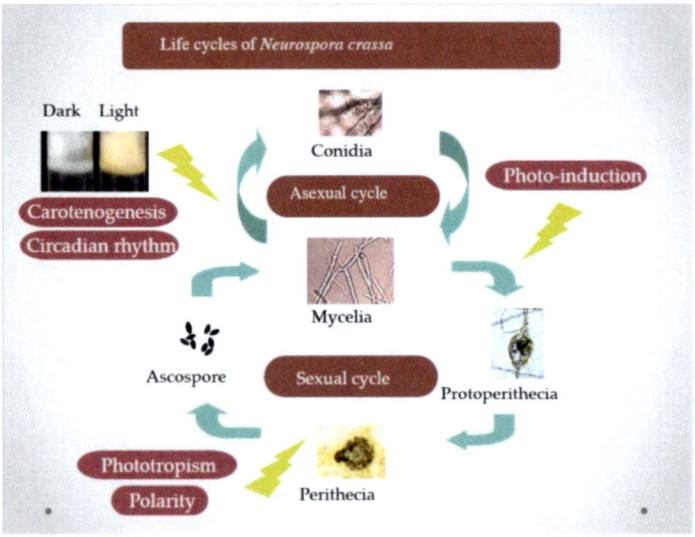

Figure 1.2.1. Life cycles of *N. crassa*. Light induced phenomena are indicated by brown circles.

The above-described phenomena are largely dependent on the presence of wild-type WC-1/WC-2. WC-1 contains FAD, and is partially dependent on riboflavin. The appearance of these phenomena in the life cycles of *N. crassa* is presented in Figure 1.2.1.

1.3. BLUE LIGHT-STIMULATED PHOSPHORYLATION OF THE NDPK-1

Mycelia grown for 36 hours in darkness were used for the preparation of the crude mycelial extract. The precise preparation method has been described in the methods reported by Oda and Hasunuma (1994, 1997). Two tube aliquots of the crude extract prepared from the wild-type mycelia were mixed for 20 s with a reaction mixture containing 4×10^{-9} M of carrier-free [γ-^{32}P] ATP. The mixture on ice was either illuminated under blue light for 1 s or not illuminated on ice, and 5 s after post-illumination, the reaction was stopped by adding SDS-sample buffer (Oda and Hasunuma 1994). The samples were developed by being subjected to gradient SDS-PAGE (poly acrylaminde gel electrophoresis, 5-20% sucrose gradient SDS-PAGE). The results of the autoradiography are presented in Figure 1.3.1.

Brief illumination with blue light stimulated the phosphorylation of a 15-kDa protein, which was purified and identified as nucleoside diphosphate kinase-1 (NDPK-1), and the protein was designated as NDPK-1 (Oda and Hasunuma 1994, 1997, Ogura et al. 1999) (Previously, designation of NDPK-1 was called psp and then NDK-1). The historical characteristics of the enzymatic reactions of NDPK-1 are summarized in Figure 1.3.2.

Among the WC (blind) mutants, we detected several mutants of NDPK-1 with no detectable phosphorylation of it (unpublished results, Hasunuma and Oda 1997). The NDPK-1 activities of these mutants,

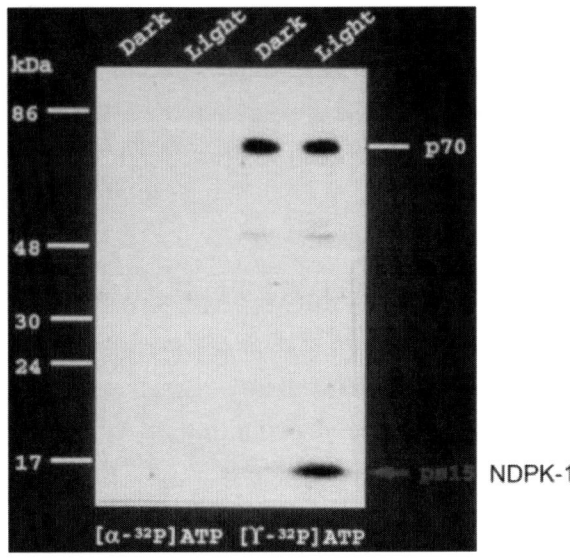

Figure 1.3.1. Blue light-stimulated phosphorylation of NDPK-1.

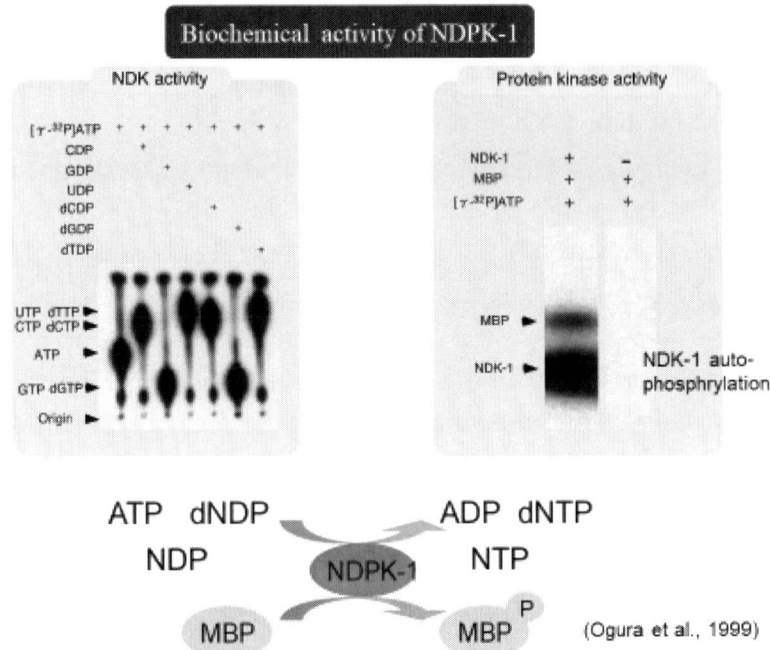

Figure 1.3.2. The historical characteristics of enzyme reactions are summarized.

FGSC # 142 (*wc-1*) and FGSC # 3817 (*wc-2*), are presented shown in Figure 1.3.3. Among them, *wc-1* (FGSC # 3628) was used for cloning of the gene, and the mutation included was NDPK-1^{P72H}, and the gene mutation was named *ndpk-1^{P72H}*. The result of the phosphorylation of NDPK-1^{P72H} is presented shown in Figure 1.3.4.

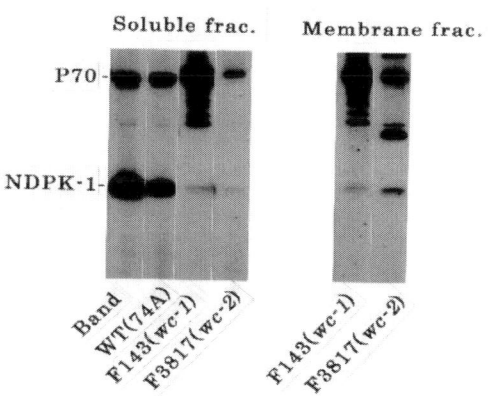

Figure 1.3.3. Phosphorylation pattern of NDPK-1 mutants in FGSC # 134 and FGSC # 3817.

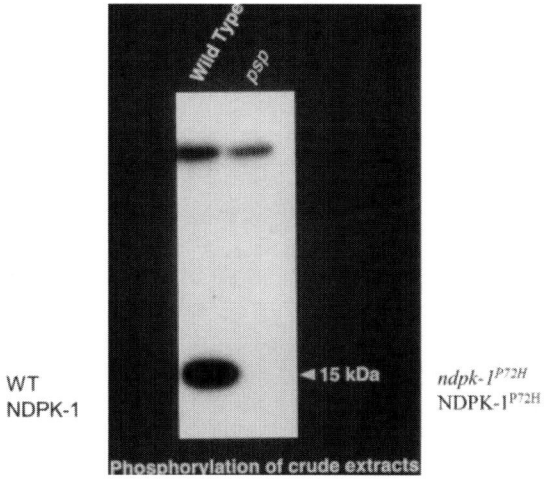

Figure 1.3.4. Phosphorylation of NDPK-1^{P72H}. The name of *psp* was changed to *ndpk-1^{P72H}*.

```
NDKC_DICDI    MSTNKVNKERTFLAVKPDGVARGLVGEIIARYEKKGFVLVGLKQLVPTKDLAESHYAEHK
Nm23H1-HUMAN  ....MA.C....I.I.....Q.....K.F.Q...R....FMQASE..LKE..VDL.
Awd-Drosoph   ....MAA......IM.....Q.....K.E.F.Q...K..A..FTWAS.E.L.K...DLS
NDK-ARATH     .......M.Q..IMI....Q...I.V.C.P.....T.K..LISVERSF..K..EDLS
NCNDK1        ...MSNQ-.Q..I.......Q....N..S.F.NR..K..AM.LTQ.GQAHL.K..EDLN
NCNDK1-P72H   ...MSNQ-.Q..I.......Q....N..S.F.NR..K..AM.LTQ.GQAHL.K..EDLN
TNK1          ...MSNQ-.Q..I--------

NDKC_DICDI    ERPFFGGLVSFITSGPVVAMVFEGKGVVASARLMIGVTNPLASAPGSIRGDFGVDVGRNI
Nm23H1-HUMAN  D....A...KYMH........W..LN..KTG.V.L.E...AD.K..T....CIQ.....
Awd-Drosoph   A....P...NYMN.....P..W..LN..KTG.Q.L.A...AD.L..T....CIQ.....
NDK-ARATH     SKS..S...DY.V.....IW...N..LTGRKI..A...A..E..T....AIDI...V
NCNDK1        TK...A...IKYMN...IC..W...DA.KTG.TIL.A........T....ALDM...V
NCNDK1-P72H   TK...A...IKYMN..HIC..W...DA.KTG.TIL.A........T....ALDM...V
TNK1          ....................A.KTG.TIL.A........T....ALDM...V

              β4▶  ◀─α4─▶
NDKC_DICDI    IHGSDSVESANREIALWFKPEELLTEVKPNPN-LYE   155
Nm23H1-HUMAN  .......EK..G...H....VDYTSCAQ.WI..      151
Awd-Drosoph   ..A....EK......NEK..V.WTPAAKDWI..       153
NDK-ARATH     .......RK......PDGPVN-WQSSVHPWVY.T      148
NCNDK1        C......N.KK..........NQWNHHSAAWIF.      152
NCNDK1-P72H   C......N.KK..........NQWNHHSAAWIF.      152
TNK1          C......N.KK..........NQWNHHSAAWIF.      152
```

Figure 1.3.5. Deduced amino acid sequences of NDPKs from various organisms, including human Nm23H1 are shown (Ogura et al. 1999).

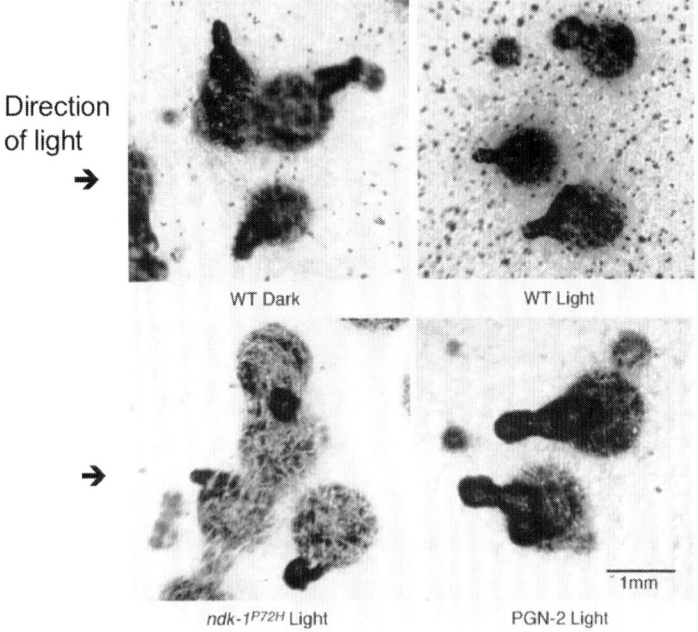

Figure 1.3.6. Assessing of the light-induced positive bending of the perithecial beak in wild-type *N. crassa*.

The deduced amino acid sequences of NDPKs are summarized in Figure 1.3.5.

The mutant was tested for the capacity to respond to lateral white light during the morphogenesis of protoperithecia to perithecia and to determine whether the mutant showed a phenotype with the light-induced bending of the perithecial beak during its formation process. We observed that the $ndpk\text{-}1^{P72H}$ mutant showed a wild-type positive response to the bending of the perithecial beak. The $ndpk\text{-}1^{P72H}$ perithecia that were formed did not allow standing upright, but instead were rolled randomly on the solid crossing medium. Therefore, the point mutation of in $ndpk\text{-}1^{P72H}$ resulted in a phenotype in which caused a defective in the perithecia, which was not able to form stand upright that did not allow the perithecia to stand (Ogura et al. 2001). This might reflect an insensitivity to gravity as shown in Figure 1.3.6.

In the mutant, $ndpk\text{-}1^{P72H}$, perithecial beaks showed light-induced bending. However, the perithecia were found to be rolling on the solid media. A genomic transformant of the wild-type $ndpk\text{-}1$ gene to the mutant, named PGN-2, showed a wild-type phenotype (Ogura et al. 2001).

1.4. LIGHT-INDUCED RELOCATION OF THE NDPK-1/CATALASE PROTEIN COMPLEX FROM THE PLASMA MEMBRANE TO THE CYTOSOL

As NDPK-1 is associated with several of protein complexes and is involved in protein localization inside the cell, we tested the light-dependent relocation of these NDPK-1 protein complexes, including NDPK-1 (Yoshida and Hasunuma 2006). Localization of NDPK-1 in the submerged mycelia, aerial mycelia, conidia, perithecia, and ascospores is presented shown in Figure 1.4.1.

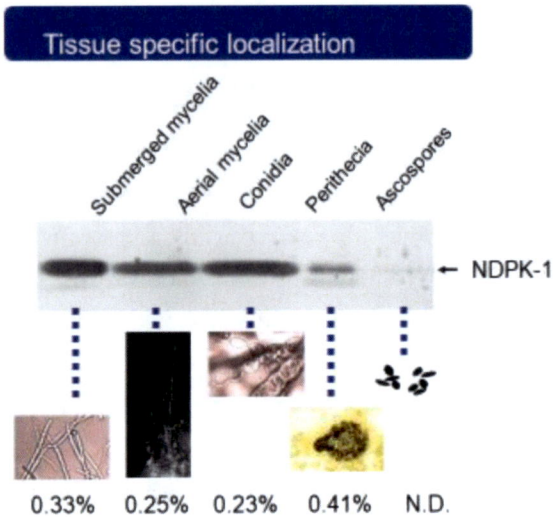

Figure 1.4.1. Tissue-specific localization of NDPK-1. The amount of NDPK-1 protein was estimated by using Western blot analysis.

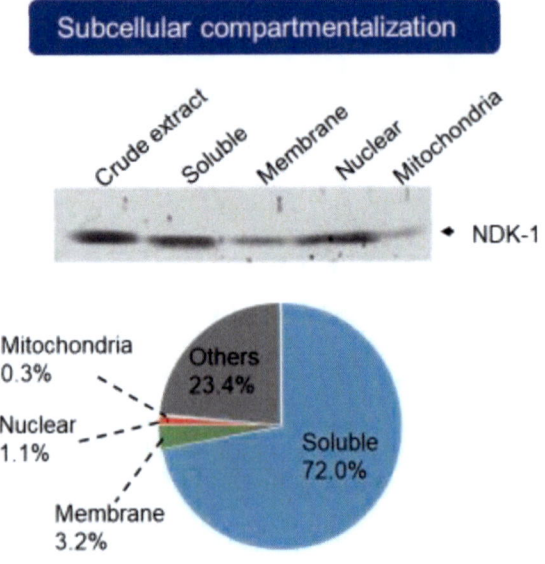

Figure 1.4.2. Subcellular compartmentalization of NDPK-1 protein in the wild-type mycelia. After subjecting proteins to SDS-PAGE, the amount of NDPK-1 proteins was estimated by using Western blotting.

Functions of the Nucleoside Diphosphate Kinase (NDPK-1) ...

The subcellular compartmentalization of NDPK-1 in the wild-type mycelia was confirmed by using Western blotting after determining the weight of proteins extracted from the mycelia. Proteins from the crude extract, and soluble fraction, membrane fraction, nuclear fraction, and mitochondrial fractions were subjected to SDS-PAGE after the protein amounts were determined. After the proteins were transferred to nitrocellulose membrane filters, the membranes were subjected to Western blotting. The results are shown in the Figure 1.4.2.

Under dark conditions, the localization of NDPK-1 in the mycelia was detected on the plasma membrane. However, upon light illumination, the enzyme translocated from the membrane to the cytosol. NDPK protein is well known to interact with the cytoskeleton and might move along the cytoskeleton to the cytosol (Yoshida and Hasunuma 2006), as shown in Figure 1.4.3.

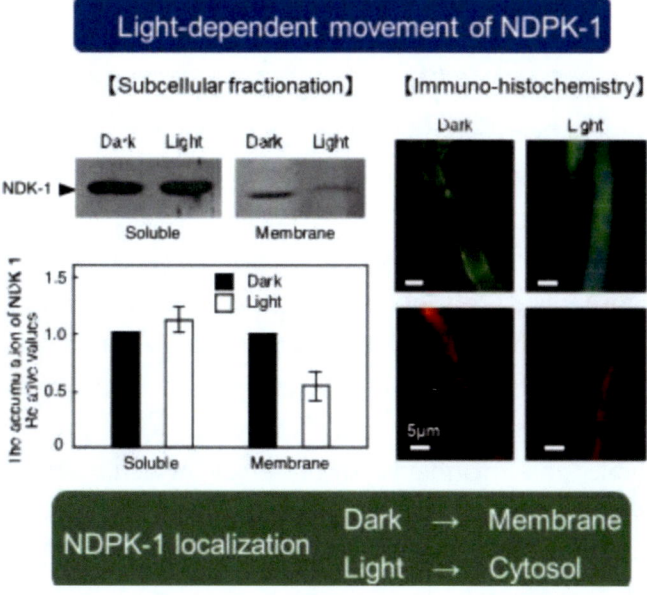

Figure 1.4.3. Immuno-histochemical representation of the light-induced re-localization of NDPK-1.

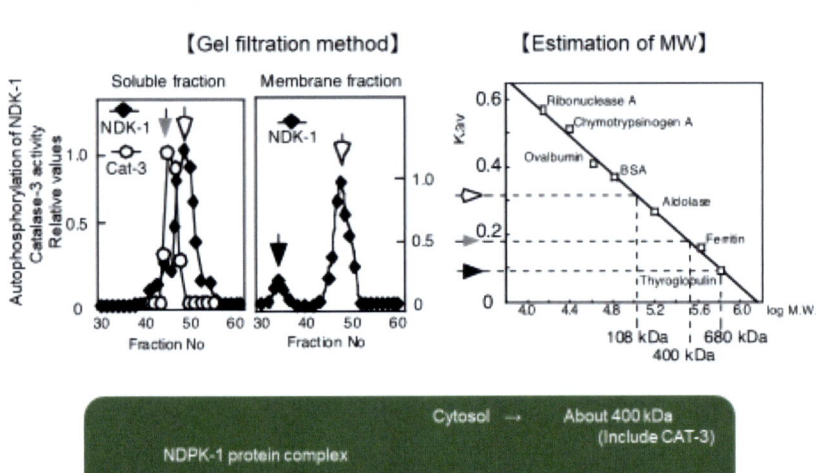

Figure 1.4.4. The protein complex of NDPK-1, protein complex which contains catalase-3.

The major cytoskeletal protein is tubulin; which is found on the plasma membranes with harboring the receptor protein (capping protein); it connects via centrosomes, along to the nucleus, constructing asters in the cytosol. The nuclei are located at the center of the asters. These results suggest that the NDPK-1/catalase complex might protect the nucleus from blue light-induced $^1O_2$ flux generated using photosensitizers such as FAD, FMN, and riboflavin by moving from the plasma membrane to and concentrating around the neighboring part of nuclear periphery, protecting it from the flux of $^1O_2$ generated by blue light.

The soluble and membrane fractions of mycelia were further prepared from the mycelia, which were subjected to SDS-PAGE to separate the proteins. After the transfer of the proteins from the gel to a membrane filter, Western blotting was performed.

Three NDP kinases have been detected in *Arabidopsis thaliana*, which are observed activities, namely, NDPK1, NDPK2, and NDPK3. NDPK1 is known to localize in the cytosol, whereas NDPK2 is to localize from the cytosol to chloroplasts, and NDPK3 is to localize from the cytosol and to mitochondria. A yeast two-hybrid system was applied to determine the functional association between the C-terminal half of NDPK1 and other proteins. Results showed that CAT1, CAT2, and CAT3 showed strong protein-protein interactions with the C-terminal half of NDPK1 (Fukamatsu et al. 2003).

To detect these interactions in *N. crassa*, the membrane and the soluble fractions of mycelia were prepared in darkness and they were subjected to molecular sieving by using gel filtration. A protein complex of approximately 400-kDa was detected in the cytosol, and this was assayed for detecting the phosphorylation of NDPK-1. Catalase-3 activity was also assayed by the activity. The membrane fraction showed a protein complex of approximately 680-kDa. The results are presented shown in Figure 1.4.4.

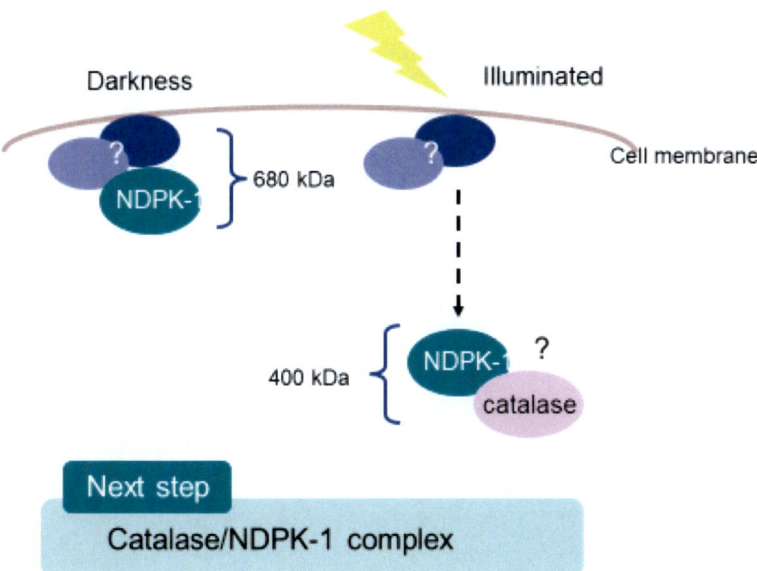

Figure 1.4.5. Light-induced relocation of a protein complex with of a molecular mass of 400-kDa; this is likely to be that the NDPK-1/catalase-3 protein complex is demonstrated. The molecular mass of NDPK-1 is estimated to be 18-kDa and is suggested to consist of six homopolymers exhibiting with a weighing 108-kDa each.

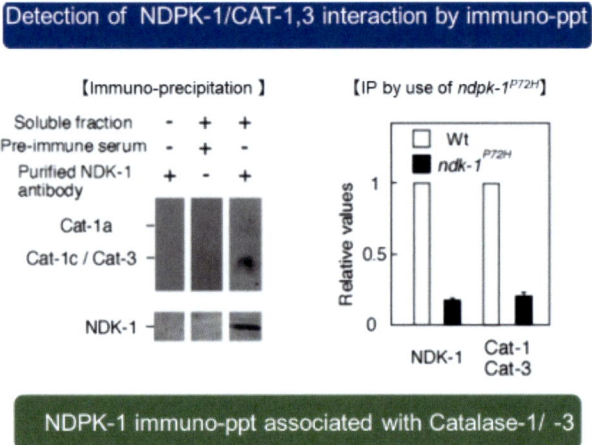

Figure 1.4.6. Immuno-precipitation of catalase-1 and/or catalase-3 using an antibody to NDPK-1. Soluble fractions from the mycelia of wild type and those from $ndpk\text{-}1^{P72H}$ mutant were used.

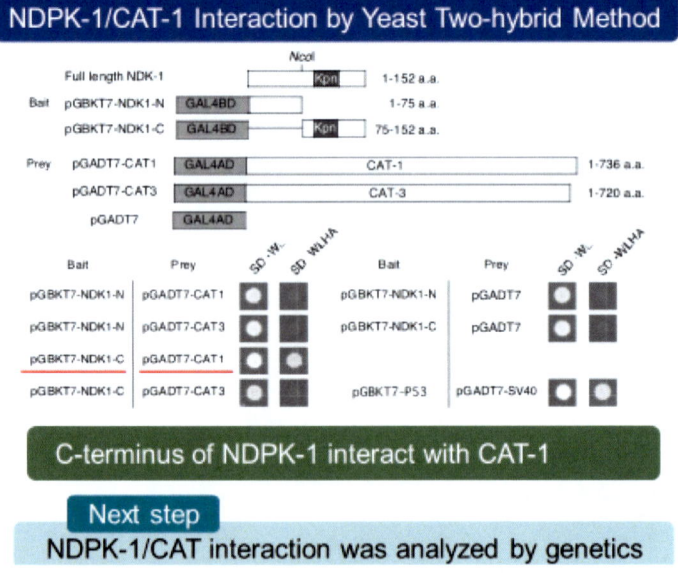

Figure 1.4.7. Yeast two-hybrid method was used to detect interaction between the C-terminal half of NDPK-1 and catalase-1. Positive interactions were observed between the C-terminal half of NDPK-1 and catalase-1. The presumed model of the molecular complex is presented shown in Figure 1.4.5. In the presence of light illumination, an NDPK-1/catalase-3 molecular complex showing a weight of approximately 400-kDa was observed.

Catalase-3 is estimated to have a molecular mass of 60-kDa and to be composed of four homopolymers exhibiting of 240-kDa each. These key proteins are estimated to be present in a 1:1 ratio in the protein of these key proteins and form individual associations within the complex.

However, we must carefully determine whether the protein complexes are composed of a single individual species or include several species of catalases. To determine the protein composition of the protein complex, we prepared the soluble fraction of mycelia from wild-type *N. crassa* and the *ndpk-1^{P72H}* mutant. These mycelial extracts were applied for an immuno-precipitation assay using an anti-body against the purified NDPK-1. The results are presented shown in Figure 1.4.6. The results indicated that the antibody to NDPK-1 resulted in the precipitation of catalase-1c or catalase-3. Using the soluble fraction from the *ndpk-1^{P72H}* mutant mycelia, only around 15% of NDPK-1^{P72H} proteins and catalase 1 and/or catalase 3 were detected.

Yeast two-hybrid method was used to detect the interactions between NDPK-1 and catalase in *N. crassa*. The results of which are presented shown in Figure 1.4.7. We could clearly detect the interactions between the C-terminal half of NDPK-1 and catalase-1. Similar results were obtained even when with the C-terminal half of NDPK-2 and catalase-1 prepared from *Pisum sativum* cv Alaska (Haque et al. 2010).

1.5. Oxidative, Light, and Heat Stresses in the Wild-Type and the *ndpk-1^{P72H}* Mutant

On illuminating mycelia with blue light, catalase-1a was strongly induced, which indicated that the region upstream of catalase-1 was methylated, and stimulated the gene expression of the gene encoding catalase-1a, which is nascent catalase-1 without any bound $^1O_2$. In the case of *ndpk-1^{P72H}*, almost no induction of catalase-1 was detected. Light illumination of the mycelia of the *ndpk-1^{P72H}* mutant did not induce the induction of catalase-1 was detected. These results indicated that NDPK-1 is well known to function as a transcription factor, and might function to stimulate the transcription of the catalase-1 gene. NDPK-1 was well phosphorylated after illumination of the crude extract. However, NDPK-1^{P72H} remained unphosphorylated, indicating that losing its enzymatic characteristics, the function of this protein may be lost. These results are presented shown in Figure 1.5.1. Loss of NDPK-1 phosphorylation of the ndpk-1^{P72H} mutant, resulted in the loss of transcription induction of catalase-1.

The capacity to induce catalase-3 activity was compared between wild-type N. crassa and the ndpk-1^{P72H} mutant under oxidative stress, exposure to 1 mM methyl viologen (MV, paraquat), and heat (42 °C) stress, treating at 42 °C. The rate of induction of catalase-3 was reduced to 50% after MV exposure. In the case of heat treatment at 42°C, the rate of reduction of catalase-3 was 60%, which as shown in Figure 1.5.2.

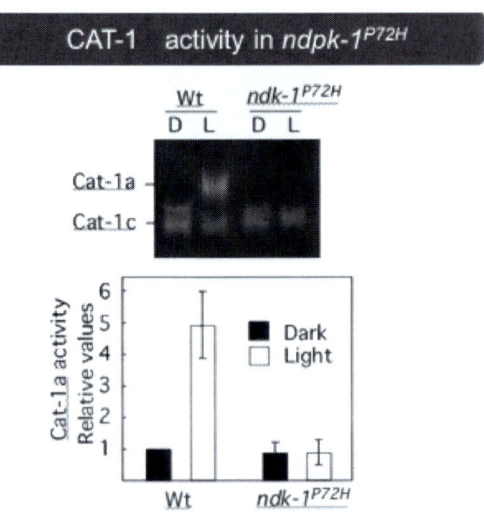

Figure 1.5.1. Effect of blue light on the mycelia of wild-type N. crassa and the ndpk-1^{P72H} mutant with respect to the catalase induction of catalase-1.

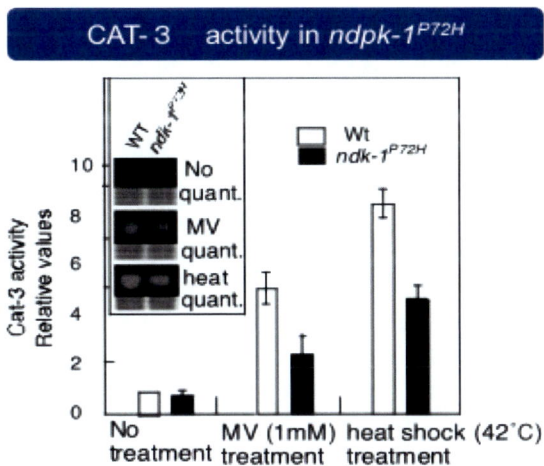

Figure 1.5.2. Comparison of catalase-3 induction between wild-type *N. crassa* and the *ndpk-1^{P72H}* mutant. The results obtained under oxidative stress with 1 mM MV and heat stress at 42 °C were compared.

A direct demonstration that NDPK-1 can bind to NADH, but the *ndpk-1^{P72H}* mutant had no ability to bind NADH. The demonstration was performed using His-tagged NDPK-1 and His-tagged NDPK-1^{P72H}. The results that are shown in Figure 1.5.3 demonstrated that NDPK-1 was bound to NADH, but NDPK-1^{P72H} did not bind to it (Wang et al. 2007a).

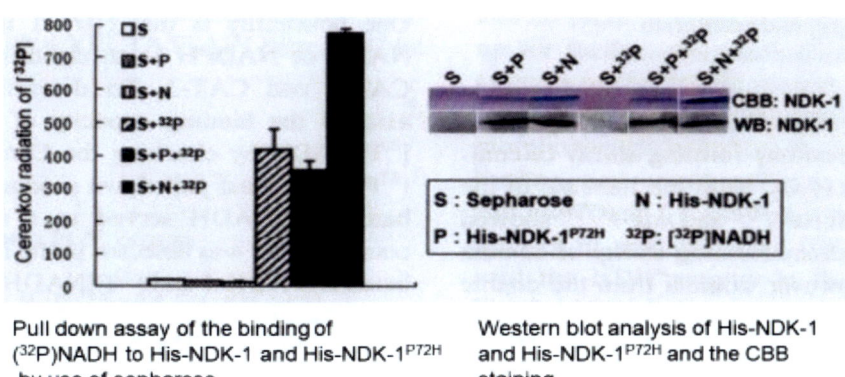

Figure 1.5.3. Binding of [^{32}P] NADH to His-tagged NDPK-1 and His-tagged NDPK-1^{P72H}.

Based on the phenomena described above, we deduced a model regarding the detoxification of $^1O_2$ (Hasunuma et al. 2011), which is shown in Figure 1.5.4.

Furthermore, we determined the effect of oxidative stress and heat stress on wild-type *N. crassa* and the *ndpk-1^{P72H}* mutant, as well as on the superoxide dismutase mutant *sod-1*. The *ndpk-1^{P72H}* mutant and the *sod-1* mutants were very sensitive to MV (paraquat), indicating that their mutations were closely related to the detoxification of singlet oxygen ($^1O_2$) to superoxide (O_2^-). These mutants also showed sensitivity to hydrogen peroxide (H_2O_2). The very *ndpk-1^{P72H}* mutant's extreme sensitivity to MV shown by *ndpk-1^{P72H}* was significantly reduced by transforming the mutant with a cDNA with a transcription initiation component. PCN-1 and the genomic DNA transformant are shown as DN. However, the recovery of the sensitivity of these mutants to MV was limited.

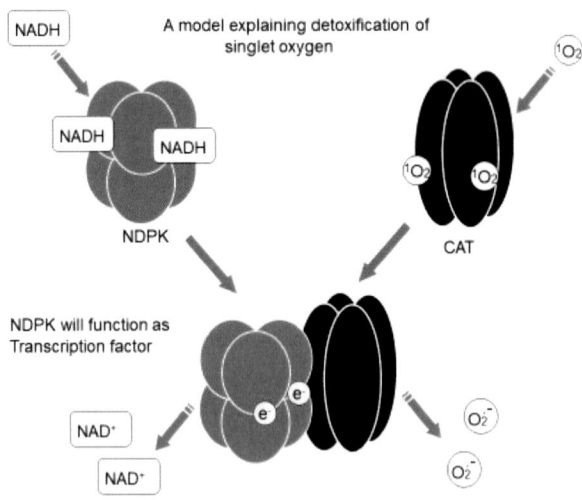

Figure 1.5.4. A molecular model explaining the process of detoxification of singlet oxygen ($^1O_2$) to superoxide (O_2^-).

Functions of the Nucleoside Diphosphate Kinase (NDPK-1) ... 19

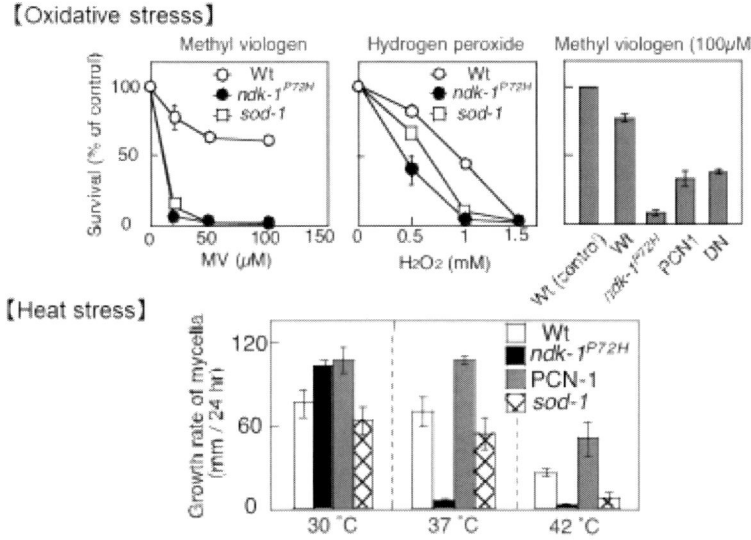

Figure 1.5.5. Comparison of oxidative stresses and heat stresses in wild-type and the *ndpk-1^P72H*, PCN-1, and *sod-1* mutants.

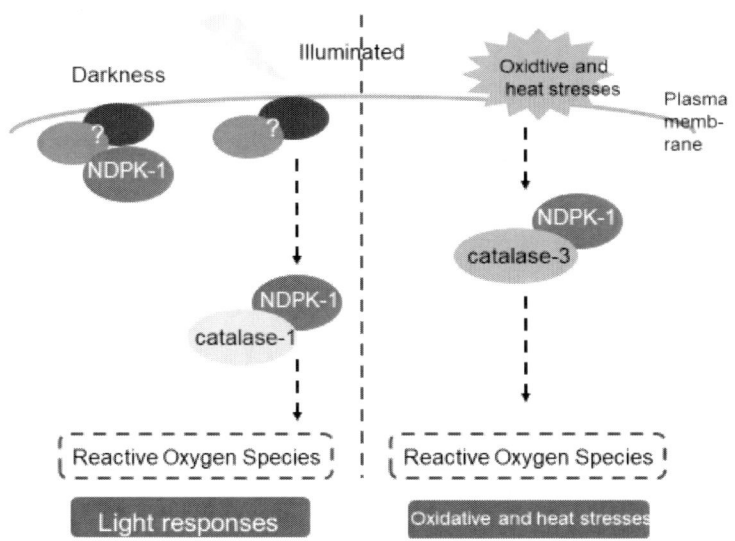

Figure 1.5.6. Possible differences caused by in light stress, to oxidative stress, and heat stresses during the formation of protein complexes between the NDPK-1/catalase-1 and NDPK-1/catalase-3.

The sensitivity to heat stress of wild-type *N. crassa*, and *ndpk-1^{P72H}*, PCN-1, and *sod-1* mutants to heat stress were compared providing the heat treatment at 30°C, 37°C, and 42°C. Although PCN-1 showed a more resistant phenotype than the wild type organism, the *ndpk-1^{P72H}* and *sod-1* mutants showed much higher sensitivity to heat stress. At 42°C, the sensitivity of *sod-1* to heat was similar to that of *ndpk-1^{P72H}*. These results are presented shown in Figure 1.5.5.

A summary of the information about effect of these stresses is shown in Figure 1.5.6. Light stress induced the movement of NDPK-1/catalase-1 complexes from the plasma membrane to the cytosol in response to ROS. However, in the case of oxidative and heat stresses, NDPK-1/catalase-3 seemed appeared to constitute the major protein complex.

1.6. The Presence of $^3O_2$ Is Required for the Inducing Carotenoid Synthesis

To investigate the molecular mechanism of photo-morphogenesis, which results in the emission of $^1O_2$, the mycelia grown on a membrane on an agar plate were illuminated in the absence or presence of air, $^3O_2$, N_2 or CO_2 gas. As shown in Figure 1.6.1, the accumulation of carotenoids in the mycelia was completely dependent on the presence of air or $^3O_2$ and the replacement of air with N_2 or CO_2 gas prevented the induction of carotenoid synthesis (Iigusa et al. 2005).

The results showed that, $^3O_2$ gas stimulated higher accumulation of carotenoids than that stimulated by air. The replacement of air with N_2 or CO_2 gas completely suppressed the accumulation of carotenoids.

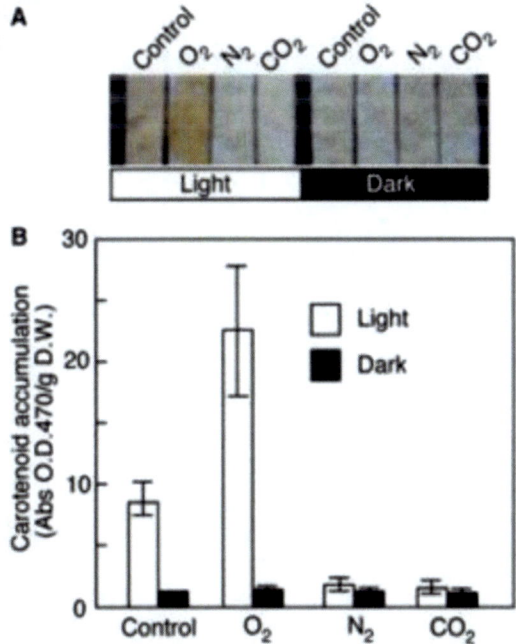

Figure 1.6.1. Accumulation of carotenoids in the mycelia exposed to light or in those maintained under dark conditions in the presence of air, $^3O_2$, N_2 or CO_2 gas.

When mycelia grown in a solid medium were subjected to light illuminated, the induction of carotenoid accumulation was observed. When the culture was immersed in a liquid medium, the induction of carotenoid synthesis was reduced significantly. However, when the liquid medium contained H_2O_2, light stimulation considerably enhanced the carotenoid accumulation, as shown in Figure 1.6.2.

We determined that in the presence of H_2O_2 in the liquid medium, the asters composed of alpha- and beta-tubulin, that formed in the mycelia were broken and disrupted. The nuclei were not protected by the aster system and were exposed to light-induced singlet oxygen atoms ($^1O_2$), which could have changed the methylation pattern of CpG islands upstream of the carotenoid synthetic genes, such as *al-1*, *al-2* and *al-3*. The methylation of CpG islands associated with these genes might be related to their induction.

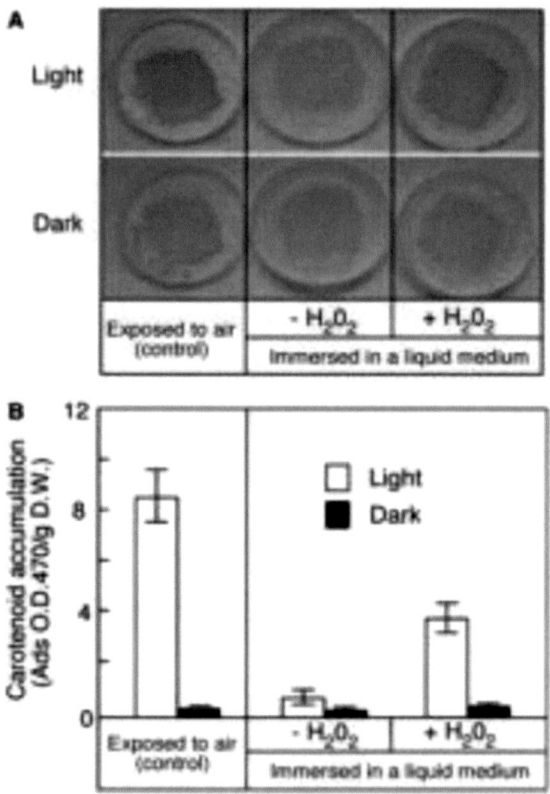

Figure 1.6.2. Accumulation of carotenoids in mycelia grown on a solid medium in the presence of air (control), with or without light illumination. The mycelial culture was immersed in a liquid medium with or without light illumination. Further, the mycelial culture was immersed in the liquid medium with or without exposure to H_2O_2, under illuminated or dark conditions.

These phenomena were further analyzed by assessing the accumulation of the *al-1* (*albino-1*) mRNA, accumulation for *al-1* (*albino-1*), which encodes a carotenoid biosynthetic enzyme. Exposure to air significantly enhanced the induction of *al-1* mRNA accumulation. However, when the mycelia were immersed in a liquid medium, mRNA accumulation was significantly reduced. When the medium was supplemented with H_2O_2, the level of *al-1* mRNA induced was more than twice of that usually observed level. These results are presented shown in Figure 1.6.3.

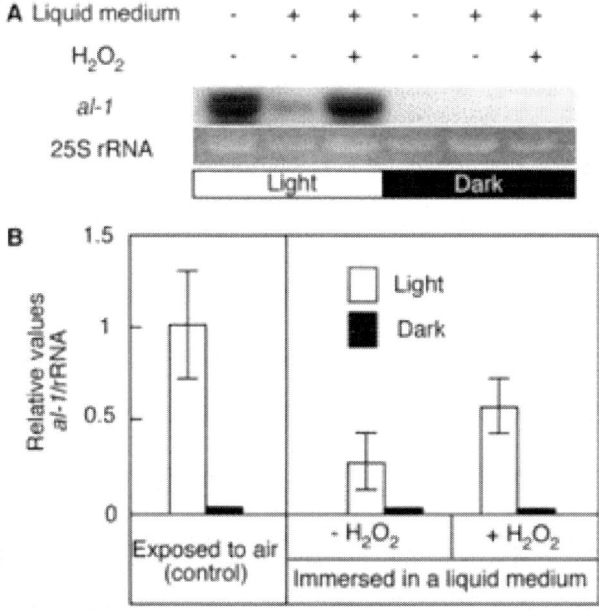

Figure 1.6.3. Presence of H_2O_2 in a liquid culture medium induced the accumulation of *al-1* mRNA.

When the culture was grown on a solid medium and was exposed to air, light illumination exposure significantly enhanced the accumulation of *al-1* mRNA accumulation. When mycelia were cultured on a solid medium in the presence of O_2 and were illuminated, the accumulation of *al-1* mRNA was increased to twice of the usually observed level. In particular, when the culture was exposed to N_2 gas and light illumination, the level of enhancement was almost equivalent to the level of mRNA accumulation observed. One possible explanation for this phenomenon could be that mycelia were cultured in the presence of O_2 and to some extent the O_2 remained in the mycelia, even though air had been replaced by N_2 gas. The purging of O_2 in the mycelia in the presence of N_2 gas might not be sufficient. Translation of the mRNA for enzyme synthesis and accumulation of carotenoids requires more ATP molecules, which will subsequently require more $^3O_2$ to be present in the mitochondria. Results are presented shown in the Figure 1.6.4.

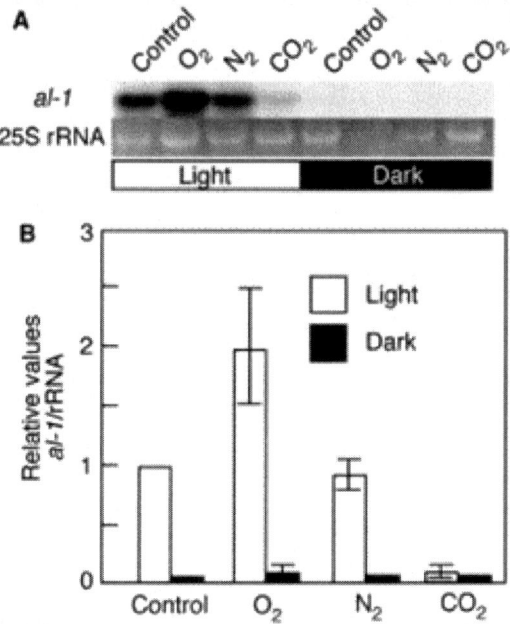

Figure 1.6.4. Accumulation of *al-1* mRNA in mycelia grown on solid media with or without light illumination, in the presence of air, O_2, N_2 or CO_2.

1.7. THE NDPK-1 FUNCTION WAS INVESTIGATED BY USING THE REPEAT INDUCED POINT MUTATION (RIP) METHOD TO INDUCE THE NDPK-1 KNOCKOUT MUTATIONS

The function of NDPK-1 was further investigated by using gene knock out created, using the repeat induced point mutation (RIP) method. We obtained two mutants. One of the mutants, designated as *ndpk-1^{RIP-1}*, showed no NDPK-1 enzyme activity and no detectable mRNA, whereas the other mutant designated as *ndpk-1^{RIP-2}* yielded a truncated protein (Lee et al. 2006, 2009). The morphology of each strain is shown in Figure 1.7.1.

Functions of the Nucleoside Diphosphate Kinase (NDPK-1) ... 25

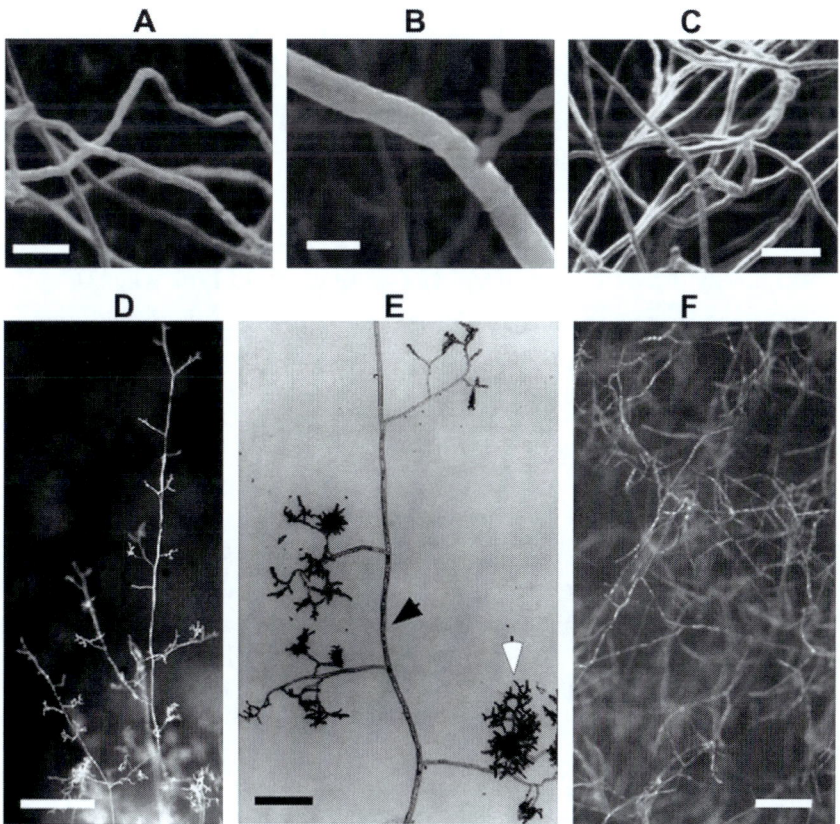

Figure 1.7.1. A: Wild-type thin mycelia, B: wild-type thick mycelia, C: *ndpk-1^{RIP-1}* mycelia, D: wild-type thin aerial hyphae with conidia, E: wild-type thick aerial hyphae (closed arrow) with macroconidia (open arrow), and F: *ndpk-1^{RIP-1}* aerial hyphae with microconidia.

This is the typical pattern of morphogenesis in wild-type mycelia and *ndpk-1^{RIP-1}* mutant mycelia.

The catalase activities in the soluble fractions of wild-type and the *ndpk-1^{RIP-1}* mutant were subjected to analyze using native-polyacrylamide gel electrophoresis (PAGE), followed by enzyme assays. In (A), *cat-3* was over expressed in the *ndpk-1^{RIP-1}* mutant. In (B), the abundance of mRNA for catalase-3 was six-times higher in the mutant than that observed within the wild-type mycelia, as shown in Figure 1.7.2, A and B.

The extension in the relative rate of growth of wild-type mycelia and the $ndpk\text{-}1^{RIP\text{-}1}$ mutant mycelia on solid media containing various concentrations of MV (methyl viologen, paraquat) and hydrogen peroxide (H_2O_2) were compared. In both cases, the relative rates of growth of the $ndpk\text{-}1^{RIP\text{-}1}$ mutant were higher when illuminated by blue light (C and D). The relative rate of growth of the $ndpk\text{-}1^{RIP\text{-}1}$ mutant was approximately three times higher than that of the wild-type when 0.5 mM MV was used. In the presence of 5 mM H_2O_2, the relative growth rate of the $ndpk\text{-}1^{RIP\text{-}1}$ mutant was approximately twice that of the wild-type. The $ndpk\text{-}1^{RIP\text{-}1}$ mutant showed thick mycelia in the presence of 0.5 mM MV and 5 mM H_2O_2 (E, closed arrow).

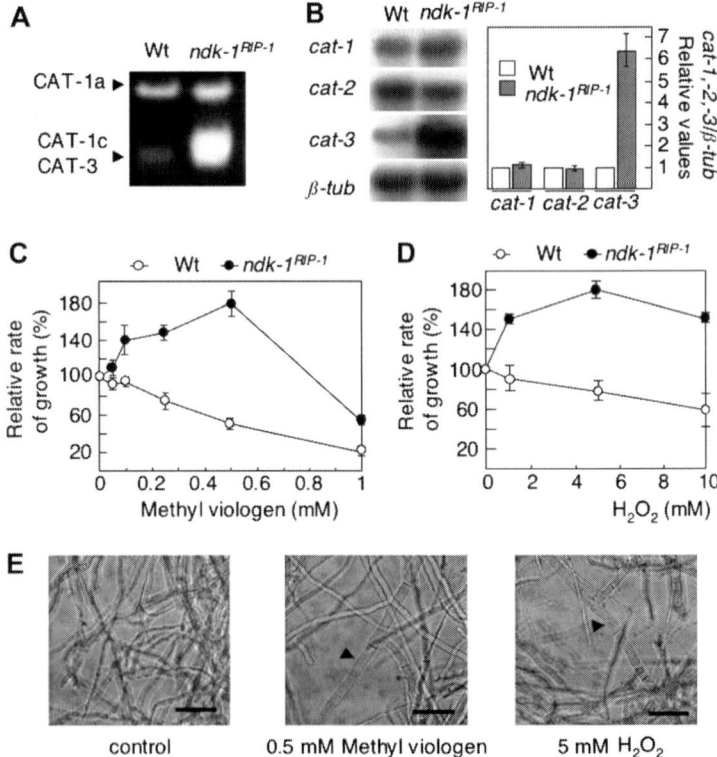

Figure 1.7.2. The effect of knocking out of *NDPK-1*: (A) Comparison of the wild-type and (B) the $ndpk\text{-}1^{RIP\text{-}1}$ mutant organisms, with respect to their growth characteristics under various conditions, including on solid media containing MV (C) or H_2O_2 (D).

In the presence of MV and H_2O_2, the $ndpk\text{-}1^{RIP\text{-}1}$ mutant nuclei in the mycelia were thoroughly exposed to singlet oxygen ($^1O_2$). As high levels of ROS in mycelial cells disrupted the aster systems and severed by the strong presence of ROS in the mycelial cells, the protein complexes of NDPK-1/catalase-1, -2, or -3 were unable to function as blocking agents, even though catalase-3 was over expressed.

The deletion of catalase-3, which is over expressed in the $ndpk\text{-}1^{RIP\text{-}1}$ mutant, was further examined. As shown in Figures 1.7.3 A and B, a deletion caused in the gene encoding catalase-3 in the $ndpk\text{-}1^{RIP\text{-}1}$ mutant recovered the full normal growth rate to return to the normal level. This phenomenon could be attributed to the overexpression of catalase-3 in the $ndpk\text{-}1^{RIP\text{-}1}$ mutant, which may block the binding of NADPH to catalase-1 and catalase-2, indicating that catalase-3 might not bind to NADPH. Catalase-1 and catalase-2 molecules bind to NADPH and functioned to maintain the normally observed ROS levels, whereas the $ndpk\text{-}1^{RIP\text{-}1}$ mutant found it difficult to detoxify $^1O_2$.

In the presence of MV and also H_2O_2, the $ndpk\text{-}1^{RIP\text{-}1}$ mutant nuclei in the mycelia are exposed to strong singlet oxygen ($^1O_2$) under blue light illumination. This is because the aster systems are disrupted by strong high levels of ROS in the mycelial cells and no blocking protein complex of NDPK-1/catalase-1, -2 or -3 complex will function even normally although the inhibitory catalase-3 was over expressed.

Catalase was reported in human to bind to NADPH, which may not be so otherwise functioning to detoxify singlet oxygen ($^1O_2$) (Kirkman et al. 1987). Under these conditions, the genomic DNA of *N. crassa*, especially the CpG islands, will be heavily methylated and circumstance-responsive genes with upstream of CpG islands will not function to sense the environmental changes of circumstances. Finally, only growth-supporting house keeping genes will function to support rapid growth. This situation may be very similar to those observed in human malignant cancerous cells.

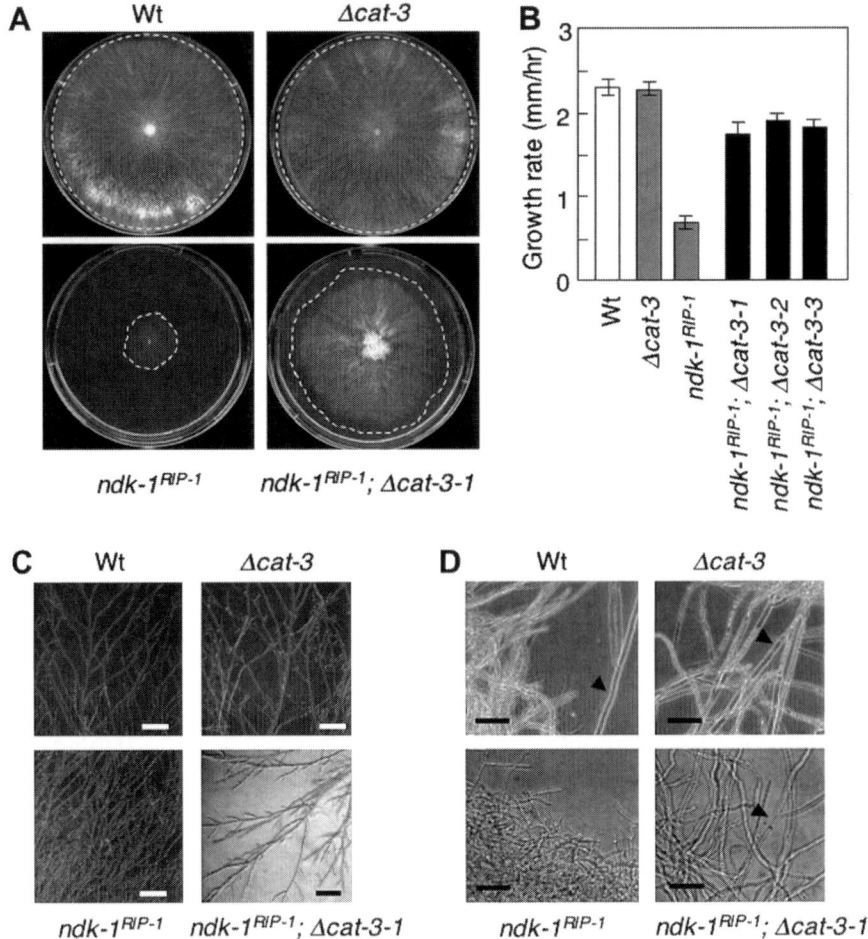

Figure 1.7.3. The functions of NDPK-1 and catalase-1, -2, and -3 were determined by obtaining in an *ndpk-1^{RIP-1}* mutant, and under the conditions of over expression, catalase-3 was also deleted to test its function (A and B). The growth patterns of the following strains on the solid medium (C) and in liquid medium (D) were observed: wild-type, catalase-3 deleted (delta cat-3) mutant, the *ndpk-1^{RIP-1}* mutant, delta cat-3-1: *ndpk-1^{RIP-1}*.

REFERENCES

Antequera, F. and Bird, A. 1993. Number of CpG islands and genes in human and mouse. *Proc. Natl. Acad. Sci.* USA. 90; 11995-11999.

Cerda, S. and Weitzman, S. A. 1997. Influence of oxygen radical injury on DNA methylation. *Mutation Research/Reviews in Mutation Research.* 386(2): 141-152.

Fritz, B. J., Kasai, S. and Matsui, K. 1989. Free cellular riboflavin is involved in phase shifting by light of the circadian clock in *Neurospora crassa. Plant Cell Physiol.* 30(4): 557-564.

Fukamatsu, Y., Yabe, N. and Hasunuma, K. 2003. Arabidopsis NDK-1 is a component of ROS signaling by interacting with three catalases. *Plant Cell Physiol.,* 44: 982-989.

Hamada, T. and Hasunuma, K. 1994. Phytochrome mediated light signal transmission to the phosphorylation of proteins in the plasma membrane and the soluble fraction of etiolated pea stem sections. *J. Photochem. Photobiol., B: Biol.* 24: 163-167.

Haque, Md. E., Yoshida, Y. and Hasunuma, K. 2008. Paraquat-resistant mutant lines in *Pisum sativum* cv Alaska: biochemical and phenotypic characterization. *Plant Biotech. Rep.,* 2: 21-31.

Haque, Md. E., Yoshida, Y. and Hasunuma, K. 2010. ROS play an important role in the plant growth and production in ROS-resistant *Pisum sativum* cv. Alaska. *Planta,* 232: 367-382.

Hasunuma, K. 2017. Detoxification of Singlet Oxygen: raising up crop yield and the clinical application, *Advances in Medicine and Biology.* Chapter 5, Vol. 121, Ed. Leon V. Berhardt, Nova Science Publishers, Co., Ltd., NY. pp115 - 132.

Hasunuma, K. 2002. 6.53.0. (3.6) *Genetics and Molecular Biology.* UNESCO-EOLSS pp. 479-504.

Hasunuma, K. 1991. Molecular mechanism of light signal perception in plants and fungi. *Trends in Photochem. Photobiol.* 1: 311-319.

Hasunuma, K., Haque, Md. E., Miyoshi, O. and Yoshida, Y. 2015. Characterization of an ROS resistant high yielding mutant *R3-1* of *Pisum sativum* cv Alaska with high temperature resistant phenotype. In *Pisum sativum*: *Cultivation, Functional Properties and Health Benefit*. Ed. Shannell Becket, Nova Science Publishers Inc., NY. pp. 55 - 75.

Hasunuma, K. and Yabe, N. 2002. 6.53.3.5. Heredity and environment; light signal transduction in plants and fungi. *On HP of EOLSS*. (also printed in the Encyclopedia).

Hasunuma, K., Yabe, N., Yoshida, Y., Ogura, Y. and Hamada, T. 2003. Putative functions of NDP kinases in plants and fungi. *J. Bioener. Biomem.* 35: 57- 65.

Hasunuma, K., Yoshida, Y., Haque, Md. E., Wang, N., Fukamatsu, Y., Miyoshi, O. and Lee, B. 2011. Global warming, plant paraquat resistance, and light signal transduction through nucleoside diphosphate kinase as a paradigm for increasing food supply. *Naunyn-Schmidberg's Arch. Pharmacol.*, 384 (4 - 5): 391- 395.

Hasunuma, K., Yoshida, Y. and Haque, Md. E. 2012. Molecular basis of signal transduction of high intensity light via nucleoside diphosphate kinase (NDPK) in *Neurospora crassa* and *Pisum sativum* cv Alaska. *Photoreceptors: Physiology, Types and Abnormalities*, Eds. Akutagawa, E. and Ozaki, K. Nova Science Publishers, Inc., NY. pp. 149-162.

Hasunuma, K., Yoshida, Y., Haque, Md. E., Fukamatsu, Y., Terajima, Y. and Matsuoka, M. 2013. Development of a method to induce ROS resistant high yielding mutant lines of sugar cane, *Saccharum officinarum* cv NiF8 and NiTn18. In *Carotenoids: Food Sources, Production and Health Benefits*. Ed. Masayoshi Yamaguchi, Nova Science Publishers, Inc., NY. pp. 79-92.

Hasunuma, K., Yoshida, Y., Kubo, M., Miyoshi, O., Nomura, K. and Haque, Md. E. 2014. Isolation of high-yielding paraquat-resistant lines of Hordeum vulgare cv Fiber Snow: Phenotype characterization. In *Barley: Physical properties, Genetic Factors and*

Environmental Impacts on Growth. Ed. Kohji Hasunuma, Nova Science Publishers, Inc., NY. pp. 219-236.

Hasunuma, K., Yoshida, Y., Matsuya, H., Nomura, K., Miyoshi, M. and Haque, Md. E. 2013. Isolation and partial characterization of reactive oxygen species (ROS) resistant mutants with high yielding in *Oryza sativa* cv Koshihikari, In *"New Developments on Signal Transduction Research"*, Ed. Masayoshi Yamaguchi, Nova Science Publishers, Inc., NY. pp.185 - 207.

Hasunuma, K., Yoshida, Y. and Lee, B. 2005. Light signal transduction coupled with reactive oxygen species in *Neurospora crassa*, In *Light Sensing in Plants.* Eds. Wada, M., Shimazaki, K. and Iino, M. Springer-Verlag Tokyo. pp. 315-321.

Huang, G., Wang, L. and Liu, Y. 2006. Molecular mechanism of suppression of circadian rhythms by a critical stimulus. *EMBO J.* 15; 25(22): 5349 – 5357.

Iigusa, H., Yoshida, Y. and Hasunuma, K. 2005. Oxygen and hydrogen peroxide enhance light-induced carotenoid synthesis in *Neurospora crassa. FEBS Lett.,* 579: 4012-4016.

Kirkman, H. N., Galiano, S. and Gaetani, G. F. 1987. The function of catalase-bound NADPH. *J. Biol. Chem.*, 262(2): 660-666.

Lee, B., Yoshida, Y. and Hasunuma, K. 2006. Photomorphogenetic characteristics are severely affected in nucleoside diphosphate kinase-1 (*ndpk-1*)-disrupted mutants in *Neurospora crassa. Mol. Genet. Genomics* 275: 9-17.

Lee, B., Yoshida, Y. and Hasunuma, K. 2009. Nucleoside diphosphate kinase-1 regulates hyphal development via the transcriptional regulation of catalase in *Neurospora crassa. FEBS Lett.,* 583: 3291-3295.

Mercer, T. R., Dinger, M. E. and Mattick, J. S. 2009. Long non-coding RNAs: insight into functions. *Nature Review Genetics, Progress.* Vol. 10. 155-159.

Oda, K. and Hasunuma, K. 1994. Light signal is transduced to the phosphorylation of 15 kDa protein in *Neurospora crassa. FEBS Lett.,* 345: 162-166.

Oda, K. and Hasunuma, K. 1997. Genetic analysis of signal transduction through light-induced protein phosphorylation in *Neurospora crassa* perithecia. *Mol. Gen. Genet.* 256: 593 – 601.

Ogura, Y., Yoshida, Y., Yabe, N. and Hasunuma, K. 2001. A point mutation in nucleoside diphosphate kinase results in a deficient light response for perithecial polarity in *Neurospora crassa. J. Biol. Chem.,* 276: 21228-21234.

Tanaka, N., Ogura, T., Noguchi, T., Hirano, H., Yabe, N. and Hasunuma, K. 1998. Phytochrome-mediated light signals are transduced to nucleoside diphosphate kinase in *Pisum sativum* L cv. Alaska. *J. Photochem. Photobiol. B: Biol.,* 45: 113-121.

Wang, N., Yoshida, Y. and Hasunuma, K. 2007a. Catalase-1 (CAT-1) and nucleoside diphosphate kinase-1 (NDK-1) play an important role in protecting conidial viability under light stress in *Neurospora crassa. Mol. Genet. Genomics,* 278: 235 - 242.

Wang, N., Yoshida, Y. and Hasunuma, K. 2007b. Loss of catalase-1 (Cat-1) results in decreased conidial viability enhanced by exposure to light in *Neurospora crassa. Mol. Genet. Genomics,* 277: 13 - 22.

Yoshida, Y. and Hasunuma, K. 2004. Reactive oxygen species affect photomorphogenesis in *Neurospora crassa. J. Biol. Chem.,* 279: 6986-6993.

Yoshida, Y. and Hasunuma, K. 2006. Light-dependent subcellular localization of nucleoside diphosphate kinase-1 in *Neurospora crassa. FEMS Microbiol. Lett.,* 261: 64 - 68.

Yoshida, Y., Iigusa, H., Wang, N. and Hasunuma, K. 2011. Cross-talk between the cellular redox state and the circadian system in Neurospora. *PLoS ONE,* vol. 6, (12): no. e28227, pp. 1-11.

Yoshida, Y., Maeda, T., Lee, B. and Hasunuma, K. 2008. Conidiation rhythm and light entrainment in superoxide dismutase mutant in *Neurospora crassa. Mol. Genet. Genomics,* 279: 193 - 202.

Yoshida, Y., Ogura, Y. and Hasunuma, K. 2006. Interaction of nucleoside diphosphate kinase and catalases for stress and light responsses in *Neurospora crassa. FEBS Lett.*, 580: 3282-3286.

Chapter 2

FUNCTIONAL ANALYSES OF THE HUMAN (*HOMO SAPIENS*) NUCLEOSIDE DIPHOSPHATE KINASE (NDPK), THE SUPEROXIDE DISMUTASE, AND THE CATALASE

2.1. GENES ENCODING THE NM23-H1 AND THE NM23-H2 GENES ARE RESPONSIBLE FOR THE NDPK ACTIVITY

Of the 10 genes that encode proteins associated with NDPK activity, genes encoding NDPKA and NDPKB have been re-designated as Nm23-H1 and Nm23-H2. These two genes were reported to be associated with the suppression of metastasis (transfer of disease: 癌転位) of cancerous cells. However, Nm23-H1 and Nm23-H2 have not been functionally analyzed. Several studies indicated that other factors control the metastasis of cancerous cells (Kahn and Steeg 2017, Hsu et al. 2015). The results obtained by analyzing *Neurospora crassa* are summarized in Chapter 1, which explains that NDPK-1 and catalase form a functional protein complex. In the cytosol, the NADH/NDPK-1/catalase/NADPH protein complex is the functional form of NDPK-1/catalase, in which catalase can bind to singlet oxygen ($^1O_2$) and NDPK-1 can bind to catalase and NADH. The transfer of electrons from NADH to bound $^1O_2$, and then subsequently NDPK-1/catalase results in release of superoxide (O_2^-), which is the first step in detoxifying $^1O_2$.

Based on localization analyses using *N. crassa*, it was shown that under dark conditions, NDPK-1 was localized close to the plasma membrane. However, upon light illumination, the NDPK-1/catalase protein complex moved along the cytoskeleton, which is made of the capping protein comprised of alpha-tubulin/beta-tubulin, on the surface of the plasma membrane. Along alpha-tubulin/beta-tubulin the protein complex moved towards the centrosomes, which contained gamma-tubulin, and along the nucleus to protect itself from the exposure to $^1O_2$.

Flagellar mobilization was achieved via the combined action of tubulin, dynein (an NDP kinase) and kinesin in the cytoplasm; dynein is an NDP kinase (Mohri, H., founder of tubulin, Mohri et al. 2012).

However, by exposure to $^1O_2$ over the limiting level, asters in the cytoskeleton, which are composed of capping proteins on the plasma-membrane, form centrosomes along the sides of the nucleus; these rings are likely to be broken and severed by $^1O_2$ and ROS. Increased exposure to excess ROS stimulates the disruption of cytoskeletal aster systems (Schneider-Stock et al. 2014). $^1O_2$ emitted from sunlight via photosensitizers causes the direct exposure of the nuclei of the neighboring cells, resulting in a reaction in which $^1O_2$ reacts with CpG islands in the chromosomes. Finally, 8-hydroxy-deoxy-guanosine is formed, which stimulates the methylation of deoxy-cytosine to 5-methyl-deoxy-cytosine in the presence of DNA methyl-transferase, with S-adenosyl-methionine used as the methyl donor.

Functional Analyses of the Human (Homo sapiens) NDPK-1 ... 37

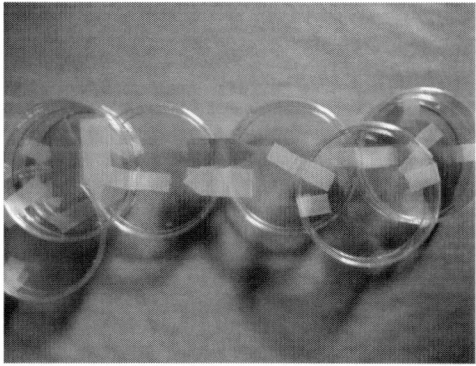

(a) Singlet oxygen $^1\Delta_g\ ^1O_2$

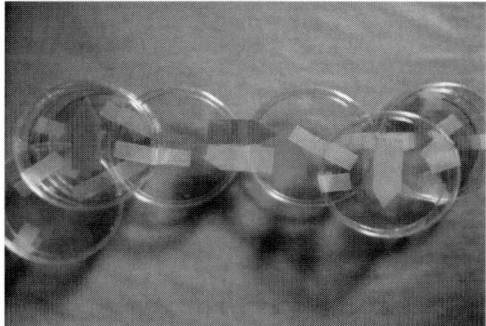

(b) Singlet oxygen $^1\Sigma g^+\ ^1O_2$

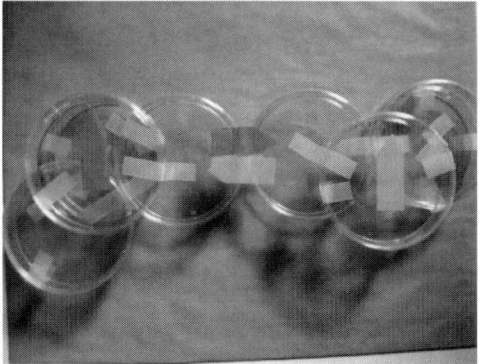

(c) Triplet oxygen $^3\Sigma g^+\ ^3O_2$

Figure 2.1.1. Excitation of $^3O_2$ to $^1O_2$ by sunlight in the presence of photosensitizers such as riboflavin, FAD (flavine adenine dinucleotide), and FMN (flavine mononucleotide), resulting in exposure of neighboring cells to emissions in the range of 200 – 500 μm. This leads to the methylation of CpG islands in the chromosomes, which alters the transcription rate of environmentally responsive genes.

Exposure of the nucleus to $^1O_2$ results in stimulation of CpG island methylation, which alters gene activation or gene inactivation to alter gene expression. Methylated CpG islands contain several functioning transcription factors, that recognize and allow these changes to occur.

Each plastic dish indicate the possible outer 4 positions of electrons, which are restricted by "Pauli's exclusion principle by the restricted two electrons with opposite +1/2, and -1/2 spin quantum number." Right side upper position is open, and therefore very reactive.

The genes encoding Nm23-H1 and Nm23-H2 are on chromosome 17 at 17p7 and, p13 (chromosome 17, short arm, position 7, and short arm, position 13). One mutation in this gene has been identified to cause aggressive neuroblastomas (Khan et al. 2015). Based on its annotation, the gene is considered as a housekeeping gene without any nearby neighboring CpG island. The typical microscopic presentation of aggressive neuroblastoma is shown in the above works.

Medical scientists mostly focus on data obtained from diseased individuals, because a medical scientist cannot perform experiments on a corresponding normal organ on account of ethical restrictions. Thus, the absence of control experiments prevent effective data from being acquired, limiting advances in "medical science". To overcome this issue, data such as DNA sequences from healthy close relatives of the patient should be compared in parallel to patient data.

After the captures of $^1O_2$ by catalase in the cytosol, electrons from bound NADH to NDPK are accepted, and $^1O_2$ is released as $O_2^{\cdot-}$. The superoxide ($O_2^{\cdot-}$) tends to accumulate because extreme exposure to too strong sunlight inevitably leads to the release of $^1O_2$ in our body via photosensitizers such as FAD, FMN, and riboflavin. As a result of it, superoxide ($O_2^{\cdot-}$) will be accumulated. Accumulated superoxide ($O_2^{\cdot-}$) can destruct and disrupts the asters, which consist of a capping protein on the plasma membranes that join alpha-tubulin/beta-tubulin to gamma-tubulin, and forming a component of the centrosomes along the sides of the nucleus. This situation is very hazardous to the nuclei of neighboring cells, as it permits the directly exposes nuclei to $^1O_2$. Therefore, understanding the high activity levels of superoxide dismutase (SOD)-mediated detoxification of $O_2^{\cdot-}$ towards triplet oxygen ($^3O_2$) and to hydrogen peroxide (H_2O_2) is essential for preventing diseases such as cancers in humans. High activity of SOD greatly increases the life span in humans. Clear proportional relationships between the life spans and SOD activities of several primate animals have been observed (Ito et al. 2007).

There are at least three types of superoxide dismutases, as shown in Figure 2.1.2.

Detoxification process of $^1O_2$ in humans
(Cu, Zn-SOD-1, Mn-SOD-2, Cu, Zn-SOD-3)

Reaction process 1 (NADPH/catalase/NDPK-1/NADH reaction)
$2\,^1O_2$ + CAT-1/NADPH + NADH/NDPK-1 $\rightarrow 2\,^1O_2$/CAT-1/NADPH + NAD^+ + $2e^-$ + NDPK-1 $\rightarrow 2\,O_2^{\cdot-}$ + CAT-1/NADPH + NAD^+ + NDPK-1

Reaction process 2 (super oxide dismutase reaction, Cu, Zn SOD-1: cytoplasm, Cu, Zn-SOD-3: inter cell space) (Mn-SOD-2: mitochondria)
Cu^{2+}, Zn-SOD-1 + $O_2^{\cdot-}$ $\rightarrow Cu^{1+}$, Zn-SOD-1 + O_2
Cu^{2+}, Zn-SOD-1 + $O_2^{\cdot-}$ + $2H^+$ $\rightarrow Cu^{1+}$, Zn-SOD-1 + H_2O_2

Reaction process 3 (catalase reaction)
NADH/NDPK-1/CAT-1/NADPH + $2H_2O_2$ $\rightarrow$ NADH/NDPK-1/CAT-1/$NADP^+$ + $2e^-$ + $2H_2O_2$ $\rightarrow$ NADH/NDPK-1/CAT-1/$NADP^+$ $\rightarrow$ $2H_2O$ + O_2 + *thermal emission (1270 nm)*

Figure 2.1.2. The $^1O_2$ detoxification processes and reaction sequences of $^1O_2$ detoxification.

(1) Superoxide dismutase-1, Cu, Zn-SOD-1, localized in the cytoplasm.
(2) Superoxide dismutase-2, Mn-SOD-2, localized in mitochondria.
(3) Superoxide dismutase-3, Cu, Zn-SOD-3, localized in intercellular spaces.

"Eukaryotic flagella and cilia" have attracted the attention of many researchers over the last century, as they are highly arranged organelles and that show sophisticated bending movements (Mohri et al. 2012). Two important cytoskeletal and motor proteins, tubulin and dynein, were first identified and described in the flagella and cilia. Half a century has passed since the identification of these two proteins, and a vast wealth of information has been accumulated regarding their molecular structures and their roles in the mechanism of microtubule sliding and bending, as well as in cell architecture. The mechanism of bending movements, and the regulation and of signal transduction in flagella and cilia has also been accumulated. This historical background and the recent advances in the field will be discussed.

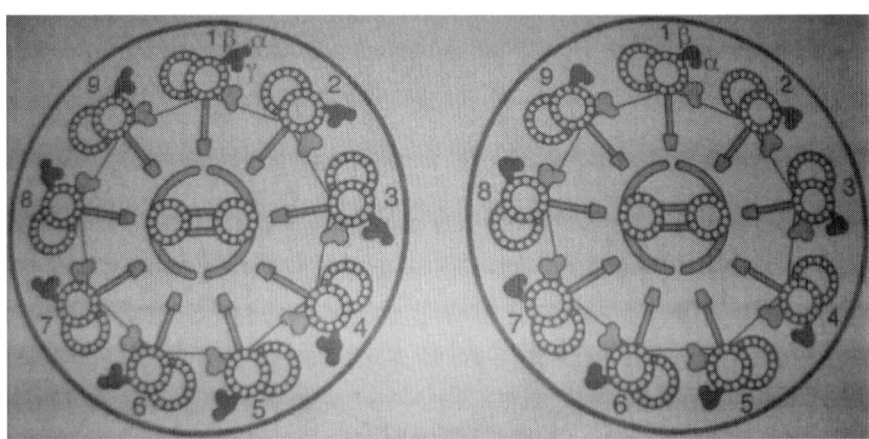

Figure 2.1.3. Schematic cross-section of a flagellum and cilium in protists and lower plants (left), and in choanoflagellates and animals (right).

Fifty years ago, the actomyosin (actin-myosin) system was considered responsible for all forms of eukaryotic motility shown by eukaryotes, including muscle contraction, amoeboid movement, cytoplasmic streaming, cell division, flagellar and ciliary movement, and axonal flow, and there was no knowledge of other systems involved in these functions. In 1945, Engelhardt described a myosin-like ATPase protein, known as "spermosin," which was obtained from bull sperm flagella. However, his group could not obtain actin. In the years following this report, many researchers investigated the presence of myosin and actin in flagella and cilia. Active ATPase activity was observed in these materials and cellular components, although the properties of ATPase in isolated flagella from marine spermatozoa were somewhat different from those of muscle myosin. However, no one had successfully isolated actin, myosin, or actomyosin from the flagella or cilia, and did not extract ATPase protein from these materials until the early 1960s.

Regarding the detailed ultrastructure of flagella and cilia, the so-called "9 + 2" structure of the flagellar and ciliary axoneme was first revealed in 1959 by Afzelius, who described the "arms" and "spokes" attaching to the outer doublet microtubules and proposed a numbering system for the outer doublets.

In the early stages of research of the cellular structure of flagellar and centrosomes along the sides of the nucleus, at least two major structures were detected. One structure showed that centrosomes consist of asters, whereas the other structure showed centrioles, which appeared to be required for structure formation as building blocks of centrosomes (Nigg and Raff 2009). After destruction of the centrosomes, centrioles can function in cellular division. Strong sunlight enhanced singlet oxygen ($^1O_2$) emission and reactive oxygen species (ROS) production, stimulating the destruction and disruption of asters in the cells and leading to cellular division. However, deregulation of centrosome numbers has been suggested to contribute to genome instability and tumor formation, and centrosomal proteins have been genetically linked to microcephaly (小頭症) and dwarfism (こびと症). Structural or functional centriole aberrations contribute to clinicopathologies, which are complex diseases that stem from the absence or dysfunction of cilia (Nigg and Raff 2009).

2.2. The Cu, Zn-SOD-1: Homodimer, Localized in the Cytoplasm, Is Encoded by a Gene on Chromosome 21 (q22.11, Long Arm, Position 22.11)

Amyotrophic lateral sclerosis (motor neuron disease：筋萎縮性側索硬化症、ルーゲーリック病) is a major disease. We selected a highly informative review article by medical doctors describing the high level of the research of amyotrophic lateral sclerosis because of the expected value of this article to the readers. Medical terms have been explained in parenthesis both in English and in Japanese (English:日本語) to facilitate understanding.

It is apparent from this review article that although transcription and the several transcription factors involved have been discussed, no attention has been given to evaluating the promoter segments of elements, which are often modified by $^1O_2$-mediated CpG methylation. This modification in several DNA elements may affect the amount and quality of mRNA, transcribed and alters the final SOD-1 enzyme activity.

For example, dioxin greatly affects processes such as sex determination in living organisms. Dioxin induces substantial productions of ROS, inducing the breakdown and disruption of the asters composed of tubulins, centrosomes, and NADH/NDPK/catalase/NADPH protein complexes. Simultaneously, this situation permits exposure of the nuclei of adjoining cells to singlet oxygen ($^1O_2$). Under such conditions, $^1O_2$ induces several types of DNA modifications, including in the CpG islands of environmentally responsive genes. ROS, including such as singlet oxygen ($^1O_2$) can causes several types of mutations genome-wide, including such as point mutations, deletions, CpG island methylation, and chromosome translocation. Mutations to occur not only in the Cu, Zn-SOD-1-encoding gene, and cause methylation of environmentally-responsive genes with CpG islands, but also change the patterns of morphogenesis, such as sex determination (Iguchi and Takasugi 1986: identified environment-disrupting compounds such as dioxin). Even in NDPK-1- and catalase-1-deficient *N. crassa*, the knocking out of the NDPK-1 and catalase-1 genes caused morphogenetic alterations in the mycelia (male organ) and non-production of the protoperithecia (female organs) (Lee et al. 2006, 2009).

As a useful reference, some of this information is presented:

Milani et al. (2011) reported a following paper: that copper, zinc superoxide dismutase-1 (Cu, Zn-SOD-1) is a detoxifying enzyme localized in the cytosol, nucleus, peroxisomes, and mitochondria. The observation that mutations in the gene encoding Cu, Zn-SOD-1 causes a subset of familial amyotrophic lateral sclerosis (FALS) cases has attracted substantial attention, with studies mainly focusing on identifying mutations in the coding region and investigations at the protein level. Considering that changes in Cu, Zn-SOD-1 mRNA levels are associated with sporadic （孤発性）ALS (SALS), the molecular understanding of the processes involved in regulating Cu, Zn-SOD-1 gene expression at the molecular level will not only reveal novel regulatory pathways governing cellular phenotypes and pathological changes, but also may reveal therapeutic targets and treatments. The review seeks to provide an overview of the Cu, Zn-SOD-1 gene structure and processes by via which Cu, Zn-SOD-1 transcription is regulated. Furthermore, the authors describe the importance of future investigating studies of post-transcriptional mechanisms and their relevance to ALS.

Glusserian et al. (2001) reported that the gene encoding the antioxidant enzyme Cu, Zn-superoxide dismutase-1 (Cu, Zn-SOD-1) is on chromosome 21q22.1, and catalyzes the dismutation of superoxide anions to hydrogen peroxide and O_2, which may lead to the increased ROS production of reactive oxygen species (ROS) in Down syndrome (DS), also known as trisomy 21 (triplicated chromosome 21 causes this syndrome (DS)). Although several studies have addressed this question and proposed the overexpression hypothesis, no specific protein-chemical data on Cu, Zn-SOD-1 protein levels in the brains of patients with DS are available.

The authors determined the protein Cu, Zn-SOD-1 and Mn-SOD-2 levels in the brains of controls (n = 9) and adult patients with DS (n = 9) and Alzheimer disease (AD; n = 9). Two-dimensional electrophoresis, followed by matrix-assisted laser desorption/ionization-mass spectroscopy-based detection and identification were conducted in the analyses.

Increased Cu, Zn-SOD-1 levels in patients with DS may reflect overexpression in the trisomic state, as a response to the oxidative stress, as has been proposed in DS by several authors. However, it well be that glial proliferation, which is markedly increased in the DS brain, may underlie the increased brain levels of this ubiquitous protein. The decrease in Cu, Zn-SOD-1 in the temporal cortex of patients with AD may reflect an antiapoptotic mechanism or simply cell loss in the brain.

2.3. THE MN-SOD-2: HOMOTETRAMER, WHICH LOCALIZES TO THE MITOCHONDRIA, IS ENCODED BY A GENE LOCATED ON CHROMOSOME 6 (Q25, LONG ARM, POSITION 25)

The binding of NADPH to catalase was also reported in humans (Kirkman et al. 1987). However, to protect catalase from the strong oxidative stresses, such as hydroxyl radicals (OH-), the strength of $^1O_2$ binding to catalase may be reduced by the donation of electrons to the bound $^1O_2$ to release superoxide (O_2^-). The major problem appears to be an unawareness of daily sunlight levels, which will inevitably cause the excitation of $^3O_2$ to $^1O_2$ on the surfaces of photosensitizers such as riboflavin, FMN and FAD which enter neighboring cells in the range of 200 – 500 μm. $^1O_2$ can be stimulated to enhance methylation of the CpG islands and regulated the gene expression. A recent study was conducted using Rose Bengal as a photosensitizer in the presence of illumination provided by a pulsed laser excited ambient $^3O_2$ to $^1O_2$, resulting in emissions in the range of 3,000 μm. The emissions were detected using a single photon detector method (Boso et al. 2016).

Mitochondria are considered as an ROS generators, with ROS produced during ATP production to overcome biotic or abiotic stresses. ATP production inevitably leads the ROS production, and mainly that of superoxide (O_2^-). Therefore, stressful life conditions increase the risk of contracting （収縮性のある） diseases and cancer development. However, whether high concentrations of cellular ROS in the cells affect the efficiency of rate of detoxification of $^1O_2$ should be considered. This may increase the rate of flux of $^1O_2$ and, in some cases, a high rate of $^1O_2$ flux may allow $^1O_2$ to enter into the nucleus, resulting in modification of deoxy-guanosine in CpG islands, which become modified to 8-hydroxy-deoxy-guanosine. This may stimulates the methylation of neighboring deoxy-cytidines to 5-methyl-deoxy-cytidines in the presence of DNA methyltransferase, with S-adenosyl-methyonine acting as a methyl donor (Xiong and Laird 1997).

Becuwe et al. (2014) reported: studied Mn-SOD-2 in breast cancer （乳がん）. Breast cancer is one of the most common malignancies of all cancers occurring in women worldwide. Predicting tumor progression is difficult because of the lack of sufficiently reliable predictive biological markers. Mn-SOD-2 may represent a rational candidate as a predictive biomarker of breast tumor metastatic progression because its gene expression is significantly altered between the early and advanced breast cancer stages, in contrast to its expression in the normal mammary gland of a normal individual. The authors report the characterization of certain gene polymorphisms and molecular mechanisms of underlying regulation of Mn-SOD-2 gene regulation. Their results improved the understanding of why the Mn-SOD-2 level is low in early breast cancer and increases in advanced stages. Several studies have demonstrated the biological significance of Mn-SOD-2 levels during proliferation and, invasive and angiogenic abilities（血管形成能） of breast tumor cells via their regulation of the superoxide anion radical ($O_2^{\cdot-}$) and hydrogen peroxide (H_2O_2) levels. Particularly, the authors have demonstrated how the mechanism by which ROS may activate some signaling pathways involved in breast tumor growth. This has led to an interesting framework for guiding translational research, suggesting ways to precisely define Mn-SOD-2 gene expression, as well as other well-known biomarkers, in addition to typical clinical parameters have been evaluated.

Krueger et al. (2016) detected a lower Mn-SOD-2 protein content in mononuclear cells, which was associated with better survival in patients treated with hemodialysis therapy. Mononuclear cell (monocyte: 単核性貪食性白血球), and hemodialysis (血液透析:半透膜を用いて血液中の不要成分を濾過する).

Mitochondrial Mn-SOD-2 converts superoxide anions to hydrogen peroxide and oxygen. Human data of the Mn-SOD-2 protein content in chronic kidney disease (CKD) patients are sparse, and the data regarding mortality data are limited and the data regarding mortality are lacking. The authors investigated the Mn-SOD-2 protein content in monocytes obtained from patients undergoing hemodialysis therapy (n = 81), those in the CKD stage 1–5 (n = 120), and healthy controls (n = 13) and conducted in-cell Western blotting assays. Mn-SOD-2

Functional Analyses of the Human (Homo sapiens) NDPK-1 ... 47

protein levels decreased from CKD stage 1 to 4, but increased again in stage 5, with and or without hemodialysis. Expression of the gene encoding Mn-SOD-2 was analyzed by quantitative real-time reverse transcription polymerase chain reaction (qRT-PCR), but no significant difference was found between the groups. Increased cellular superoxide production reduced Mn-SOD-2 protein content. This effect was abolished by the superoxide dismutase mimetic, tempol (経時的に変化する). We did not detect nitrotyrosine modifications of Mn-SOD-2 in CKD. Gel electrophoresis and Western blot analysis did not reviel nitrotyrosine modifications of Mn-SOD-2 in CKD. In patients with stage 5 CKD who were undergoing hemodialysis therapy, a higher than median Mn-SOD-2 protein content was associated with higher all-cause mortality. In conclusion, Mn-SOD-2 protein content decreased in CKD until stage 4, whereas transcription of the gene expressing Mn-SOD-2 did not. Increased cellular superoxide anion production may affect Mn-SOD-2 protein content. In patients with advanced CKD (stage 5), the Mn-SOD-2 protein content increased again, although the increased Mn-SOD-2 protein content in these patients did not confer a survival benefit.

2.4. THE CU, ZN-SOD-3: HOMOTETRAMER LOCALIZED IN INTER CELLULAR SPACES, IS ENCODED BY A GENE ON CHROMOSOME 4 (Q15.2, LONG ARM, POSITION 15.2)

The break down and disruption of tubulin-based aster structures can induce morphological changes in cancerous cells, causing malignant cancerous cells to develop a spindle-like form. These structures show the lowest efficiency in blocking the entry of $^1O_2$ into the nuclei and structures that are not protected by a plasma membrane such as the Golgi apparatus or the nuclear membrane in animal cells with low concentrations of unsaturated fatty acids. The alpha- and beta-tubulin-based structures of asters, which block the entry of $^1O_2$, leads to the formation of Nm23-H1/catalase and Nm23-H2/catalase complexes and centrosomes, which are composed of gamma-tubulin-based structures along the nuclear periphery. Excessive exposure to $^1O_2$ and other stresses leads to the accumulation of ROS, which disrupt the asters and destroy the tubulin structures, protecting the nuclei from exposure to $^1O_2$.

The Cu, Zn-SOD-3 is localized and active in the inter-cellular space. However, examination of Cu, Zn-SOD-3 function is challenging.

The author discusses the following three papers: Pedersen and Mattson (1999) analyzed Cu, Zn-SOD (-1 or -3) mutant mice, demonstrating "no benefit of dietary restriction on disease onset or progression in amyotrophic lateral sclerosis Cu, Zn-superoxide dismutase mutant mice". Amyotrophic lateral sclerosis (ALS) is a fatal disease characterized by spinal cord motor neuron degeneration, resulting in progressive paralysis （麻痺の進行）. Some cases of ALS are caused by mutations in the antioxidant enzyme Cu, Zn-SOD-1 or -3, and transgenic mice expressing ALS-linked Cu, Zn-SOD mutations (SODMutM: Cu, Zn-SOD mutant mouse) exhibit a phenotype analogous to that of human ALS patients. Dietary restriction (DR) is a well-established means of extending the lifespan in rodents, which reduce cellular oxidative stress revels. The authors evaluated whether DR can retard the development of the clinical phenotype and extend the lifespan of SOD MutM mouse (Cu, Zn-SOD mutant mouse). There was no significant difference in the age of disease onset in mice placed on a DR regimen beginning at 6 weeks of age compared to mice fed *ad libitum* (according to performer's wishes). However, the disease duration was reduced, indicating that DR accelerates the clinical course. Histological analyses indicated a similar extent of lower motor neuron degeneration in SOD MutM mice maintained on DR or *ad libitum* diets. The authors conclude that dietary manipulation, which extends lifespan, had no beneficial effects in an animal model of familial ALS.

Table 2.4.1. A comparison of the unsaturated fatty acids content in plants, humans and other animals

	Saturated g/100 g	Monoun-saturated g/100 g	Polyun-saturated g/100 g	Cholesterol mg/100 g	Vitamin E mg/100 g
Animal fats					
Lard (1)	40.8	43.8	9.6	93	0.60
Duck fat (1)	33.2	49.3	12.9	100	2.70
Butter	54.0	19.8	2.6	230	2.00
Vegetable fats					
Coconut oil	85.2	6.6	1.7	0	0.66
Cocoa butter	60.0	32.9	3.0	0	1.88
Palm oil	45.3	41.6	8.3	0	33.12
Olive oil	14.0	69.7	11.2	0	5.10
Sunflower oil	11.9	20.2	63.0	0	49.00

A comparison of the unsaturated fatty acid content in plants, humans, and other animals is summarized in Table 2.4.1. Part of this table was obtained from Wikipedia.

Based on this data, the consumption of sunflower oil has been recommended. To avoid the development of cancerous cells in the body, the ratios of unsaturated fatty acids and vitamin E content should be very high.

The unsaturated fatty acid content in plant membrane systems is high ($\geq 80\%$), which protects nuclei from direct exposure to $^1O_2$ emitted from the photosensitizer, following exposure to intense sunlight. This phenomenon was first detected by M. Yamada (Sakaki et al. 1990) (the founder of the field of a research of ozone-resistant phenotypes observed with high unsaturated fatty acid content). The ozone reaction occurred as follows:

$$2O_3 \rightarrow 2\,^3O_2 + {}^1O_2$$

Laukkanen (2016) evaluated whether extracellular SOD functions as a growth promoter or tumor suppressor. Transfer of the gene encoding this extracellular Cu, Zn-SOD-3 into damaged tissues resulted in increases healing and cell proliferation, and decrease apoptosis and inflammatory cell infiltration (浸潤). At the molecular level, *in vivo* overexpression of Cu, Zn-SOD-3 reduced superoxide anion (O_2^-) concentrations and increased mitogen kinase activity, suggesting that Cu, Zn-SOD-3 has a life-supporting function. This hypothesis is further supported by studies reporting significantly increased mortality in Cu, Zn-SOD-3 conditional knockout mice. However, among cancerous cells, Cu, Zn-SOD-3 was shown to either increase or decrease cell proliferation and survival depending on the model system used, indicating that Cu, Zn-SOD-3 associated growth mechanisms are not completely understood. The main discoveries regarding Cu, Zn-SOD-3 dependent growth regulation and signal transduction have been reviewed, which highlight that the role of Cu, Zn-SOD-3 in tumorigenesis is only partially understood. Recent studies suggested that Cu, Zn-SOD-3 has dose-dependent effects on primary tumor growth and metastatic activity, which may depend on the ROS detoxification ability in different types of tumor cells to detoxify ROS in various manners. Thus, several different approaches should be used to determine the role of Cu, Zn-SOD-3 in tumorigenesis. Most importantly, the results obtained from *in vitro* experiments showed that moderate Cu, Zn-SOD-3 mRNA over-expression induces primary cell immortalization and transformation. The mechanism underlying this phenomenon should be further examined to determine if the results of the *in vitro* experiments can be replicated *in vivo* model systems, and the mechanism underlying this phenomenon should be further elucidated. Second, high Cu, Zn-SOD-3 mRNA expression correlates with increased benign (温和な) growth, whereas low Cu, Zn-SOD-3 mRNA expression correlates with increased malignant progression; studies of the differences in signal transduction between primary and transformed cells are needed. The current hypothesis suggesting that the increased aggressiveness of cancer cells caused by decreased Cu, Zn-SOD-3 mRNA expression requires a mechanistic explanation. Furthermore, as high expression levels of Cu, Zn-SOD-3 may induces cancer cell apoptosis, it would be interesting to determine whether regulation of the gene encoding Cu, Zn-SOD-3 under certain cellular conditions enables supra-physiological expression of the enzyme to result in cellular death, Cu, Zn-SOD-3 has possesses the characteristics of a tumor suppressive characteristics. Although several studies have established the function of Cu, Zn-SOD-3 as a regulator of cellular growth, the enzyme itself may not be a suitable cancer drug or target molecule. Rather, studies of Cu, Zn-SOD-3-related signal transduction may reveal the mediators of tumor progression, which can be used as targets in preclinical and clinical studies.

Gu et al. (2013) reported the mechanisms by which omega-3 polyunsaturated fatty acids prevent progression of prostate cancer. It is well-known that omega-3 polyunsaturated fatty acids (n-3 PUFA), mainly eicosapentaenoic acid (EPA 20:5) and docosahexaenoic acid (DHA 22:6), possess health benefits. Epidemiological studies dating back to the 1970s were among the first to suggest that dietary PUFA might be beneficial for preventing disease. Even today, studies continue to demonstrate the health benefits of n-3 PUFA; however, the mechanism of action of n-3 PUFA is not completely understood. Several new observations have advanced our understanding of the activities of n-3 PUFA in human disease. For example, the DHA-receptor GPR120 was demonstrated to sense and control obesity (grow fat 肥満) and metabolic syndrome. Recently identified omega-3 mediators, resolvins and protectins, were demonstrated to possess anti-inflammatory and pro-resolving activities. The purpose of this review is to highlight recent advances in research of the mechanisms by which n-3 PUFA modulates prostate cancer development. Terms frequently used in this field are summarized in the Tables 2.4.2 and 2.4.3.

Table 2.4.2. Terms frequently used

PUFA:	Polyunsaturated fatty acid	EPA:	Eicosapentaenoic acid (20:5, n-3)	DHA:	Docosapentaenoic acid (20:5, n-3)	LA:	Linoleic acid (18:2, n-3)	AA:	Arachidonic acid (20:4, n-3)
ALA:	Alpha linolenic acid (18:3, n-3)	FADS:	Fatty acid desaturase	GLA:	Gamma-linolenic acid (18:3, n-6)	DGLA:	Dihomo-gamma-linolenic acid (20:3, n-6)	KAR:	3-Ketoacyl-CoA reductase
HACD:	3-Hydroxyl-CoA dehydratase	TECR:	Trans-2,3-enoyl-CoA reductase	DPA:	Docosapentaenoic acid (22:5, n-3)	PC:	Phosphatidylcholine	PS:	Phosphatidylserine
PE:	Phosphatidyl ethanolamine	PI:	In Phosphatidylositol	SA:	Stearic acid (18:0)	GPCR:	G Protein-coupled receptor	EGFR:	Epidermal growth factor receptor
PKC:	Protein Kinase C								

Table 2.4.3. Terms frequently used

AKT:	Serine/threonine protein kinase (protein kinase B)	PI3K:	Phosphatidyl-linositol-3-kinase	PIP3:	PI-3,4,5-trisphosphate	PH:	Pleckstrin homology	PDPK1:	Phosphoinositide-dependent kinase-1
SDC-1:	Syndecan-1	COX:	Cyclooxygenase	LOX:	Lipoxygenase	RvE1:	E-Resolvin 1	RvD1:	D-Resolvin 1
TLR:	Toll-like receptor	PPAR:	Peroxisome proliferator-activated receptor	MCFA:	Medium-chain fatty acid	BMDC:	Bone marrow-derived CD11C+macrophage	KO:	Knock out
HFD:	High-fat diet	Nrf2:	Nuclear Factor-erithroid-2-related factor 2	Keap 1:	Kelch-like ECH-associated protein 1	ARE:	Antioxidant response element	LPS:	Lipopolysaccharide

Thus, diseases result from high levels of ROS, which further reduce the detoxification rate of $^1O_2$ and cause cancerous cells to proliferate without receiving environmental information from the surrounding cells. Genes associated with 45,000 CpG islands upstream of environmentally-responsive regulatory gene elements in the haploid human genome are gradually over-methylated because of excessive stress, resulting in increased ROS generation. When nuclei are exposed to high levels of $^1O_2$, the tissues cease to respond to environmental information and proliferate limitlessly. Cells that are highly exposed to $^1O_2$ proliferate in response to the transcription of house-keeping genes without upstream CpG islands in the genome. These cells do not respond to inhibitory signals that repress proliferation generated by the environmentally-responsive genes controlled by upstream CpG islands. The total number of genes per haploid genome has been determined to be 80,000.

However, if environmental conditions, including $^1O_2$ exposure, are less severe or extreme, the cells lose the ability to vigorously proliferate, resulting a gradual loss of methylation in the region upstream of the CpG islands. CpG island methylations are not very stable; rather, the methylation status can be reversed by $^1O_2$ at a low flux rate. At a low rate of flux, $^1O_2$ enhances the transcription of noncoding RNA. In response to the presence of noncoding RNA, de-methylation of 5-methyl CpG is stimulated, although the precise mechanism of de-methylation is still under investigation.

Furthermore, slowly proliferating cancerous cells are ingested by cancer cell-eating cell systems such as the B-cell and T-cell systems.

2.5. Functional Analysis of the Catalase Encoded by a Gene on: The Catalase Localization: Chromosome 11 (p13, Short Arm, Position 13)

Human beings there possess only one catalase gene at the chromosome position, 11p13. The functions of catalase are limited only to conventional activity as described in by the following equation.

$$2H_2O_2 \rightarrow 2H_2O + O_2$$

Reports on the binding of $^1O_2$ at to the heme-group of catalase and also no information was published whether the catalase form complex between human Nm23-H1 nor Nm23-H2 are lacking. NADH binding to Nm23-H1 nor Nm23-H2 is not known. Therefore, current information regarding the $^1O_2$ detoxification capacity by a catalase-forming complex with Nm23-H1/or Nm23-H2 complex was almost negligible. Catalase and Nm23-H1, or Nm23-H2 bound with NADPH and NADH, respectively, will provide electrons to the catalase-bound $^1O_2$ with the release of superoxide (O_2^-). The fundamental process of $^1O_2$ detoxification is not yet analyzed in human beings, which will provide a very difficult situation to pose serious challenge in treating malignant cancerous cells and also even many diseases characterized by the abnormal ROS accumulation. These processes to regulate $^1O_2$ and followed by ROS production are summarized in Figure 2.5.1.

The human genome harbors several pseudo genes with no catalase activity, which may contribute to the repair of the mutated catalase-encoding gene. However, in case of catalase, the binding of NADPH to catalase is well-known, which may provide electrons to the bound singlet oxygen ($^1O_2$). These possibilities should be clarified to understand the exact detoxification process of $^1O_2$.

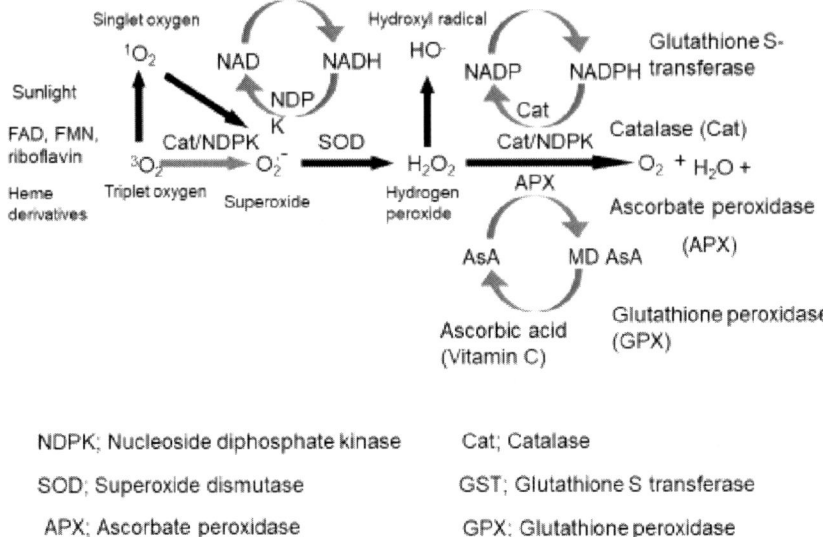

Figure 2.5.1. Evolution of $^1O_2$ by sunlight, followed by possible detoxification processes to superoxide (O_2^-) and to hydrogen peroxide (H_2O_2).

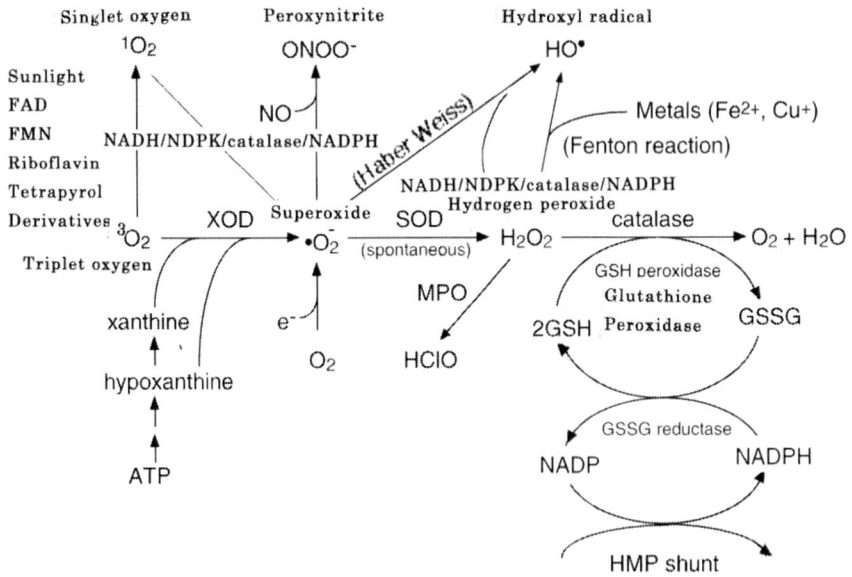

Figure 2.5.2. Detoxification process of singlet oxygen ($^1O_2$) via superoxide (O_2^-) to hydrogen peroxide (H_2O_2). The HMP shunt represents the hexose monophosphate pathway.

The effect of sunlight causing on the evolution of $^1O_2$ via photosensitizers, such as FAD, FMN, riboflavin, and derivatives of heme should be analyzed in detail. Currently, it is known that $^1O_2$ is generated by the interaction of sunlight with the photosensitizers, during which excited triplet oxygen ($^3O_2$) emits $^1O_2$ in a the range of 200 to 500 μm, a process of which is not considered in the humans beings. A similar situation will provide the origin of which can result in the onset of several diseases and permit to promote cancerous cell proliferation.

These observations were summarized in Figure 2.5.2.

I would like to introduce the following paper as it strongly suggests that upstream CpG island methylation may be a key factor for regulating the expression of the catalase-encoding gene regulation in humans. The upstream CpG island of DNA methylation may be the major factor for regulating the gene expression.

Glorieux et al. (2018) reported the research article: evaluated the potential mechanisms regulating catalase expression in breast cancer cells. The development of cancer cell resistance against prooxidant (prooxidant antioxidant balance, 酸化を促進する) drugs limits their potential clinical use. MCF-7 (macrophage chemotactic factor, 大食細胞化学走性因子) breast cancer cells chronically （慢性的に）exposed to ascorbate/menadione (precursor of synthetic vitamin K, 合成ビタミンK前駆体) became resistant by increasing mainly owing to increase in catalase activity. As catalase appears as to be an anticancer target, the elucidation of the mechanisms regulating its expression is an important issue. In MCF-7 and redox cells (cells controlling successive reduction, 電子供与過程に関わる細胞), karyotype analysis showed that chromosome 11 of these cells is not altered compared to that of healthy mammary epithelial cells. The genomic gain of catalase locus observed in MCF-7 and redox cells cannot explain the differential catalase expression (resox cells in this paper correspond to redox cells, and therefore the resox was replaced with by redox cells). As ROS cause DNA lesions, the activation of DNA damage signaling pathways may influence catalase expression. However, none of the related proteins (i.e., p53 (working to important for monitoring and healing of DNA lesion), or ChK (check point kinase 1)) were activated in redox cells compared to in MCF-7. The Abl kinase (Abelson murine leukemia viral oncogene homolog 1) may lead to catalase protein degradation via posttranslational modifications, but neither ubiquitination nor phosphorylation of catalase was detected after catalase immunoprecipitation. Catalase mRNA levels did not decrease after actinomycin D treatment in both of either cell lines. DNMT inhibitor (5-aza-2-deoxycytidine) increased catalase protein level in MCF-7 and its resistance to prooxidant drugs. Chromatin remodeling appears as the main regulator of catalase expression in breast cancer after chronic exposure to an oxidative stress. The abbreviations used are described in the Table 2.5.1.

Table 2.5.1. Additional description on the abbreviations used was made on this table

Akt/PKB:	Protein kinase B	AP-MS:	Affinity purification followed by mass spectroscopy	Arg:	c-Abl-related gene	ATM:	Ataxia telangiectasia mutated	ATR:	Ataxia telangiectasia and Rad3 related
Asc/Men	Ascorbate/menadione	c-Abl:	Abelson murine leukemia viral oncogene homolog 1	ChIP:	Chromatin precipitation	Chk:	Checkpoint kinase	DNA-PK:	DNA-activated protein kinase
DNMT:	DNA methyl transferase	FISH:	Fluorescence in situ hybridization	FoxO3:	Forkhead box O3	HDAC:	Histone deacetylase	MEF:	Mouse embryonic fibroblast
Oct-1:	Octamer-binding transcription factor 1	PAR alpha:	Retinoic acid receptor alpha	ROS:	Reactive oxygen species	TSA:	Trichostatin A	UTR:	Untranslated region
Aniridia:	Gonadoblastoma and mental retardation (syndrome)								

2.6. Mitochondrial ATP Production Is Associated with ROS Production Triggered by Cytosolic Free Ca^{2+} Concentration, $[Ca^{2+}]$cyt

$[Ca^{2+}]_{cyt}$ control is increased during the day time because of sunlight. In *Neurospora crassa*, sunlight induces the production of large amounts of singlet oxygen ($^1O_2$) via photosensitizers, thereby decreasing the integrity of the monolayer of membrane systems of the endoplasmic reticulum, which is composed of unsaturated fatty acids. Consequently, large amounts of Ca^{2+} are released in the cytosol from the Ca^{2+} storage in the endoplasmic reticulum. The released Ca^{2+} increases $[Ca^{2+}]$cyt, causing $[Ca^{2+}]$mit to increase (Hasunuma and Shinohara (1987): written in Japanese) as shown in Figure 2.6.1.

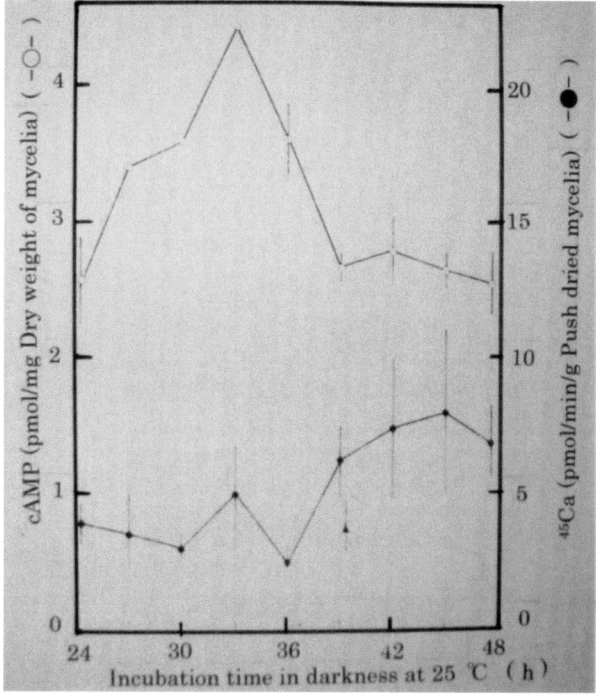

Figure 2.6.1. Circadian rhythm of the rate of incorporation of $^{45}Ca^{2+}$.

Right ordinate: $^{45}Ca^{2+}$ (pmol/min/g push dried mycelia), Left ordinate: cAMP (pmol/mg dry weight of mycelia). The conidial suspension was inoculated in 10 ml of Fries minimal liquid medium and the culture was incubated in the dark at 25°C for 12 h, after which the cultures were illuminated (60 µmol/m²/h) for 12 h. Thereafter, the cultures were kept again incubated in the dark at 25°C. Every 3 h, $^{45}Ca^{2+}$ was added to one of the culture for 10 min, and then the culture was push-dried through filter paper. After weighing the push-dried mycelial mat, the radioisotopic counting was conducted by Cherenkov counting in 5 ml of H_2O. Ten milliliters of ethanol were added to extract cAMP. After removing the mycelial mat, the extract was freeze-dried and cAMP was measured by using the YAMASA cAMP assay kit. The mycelial mat was heat-dried and the weight was measured.

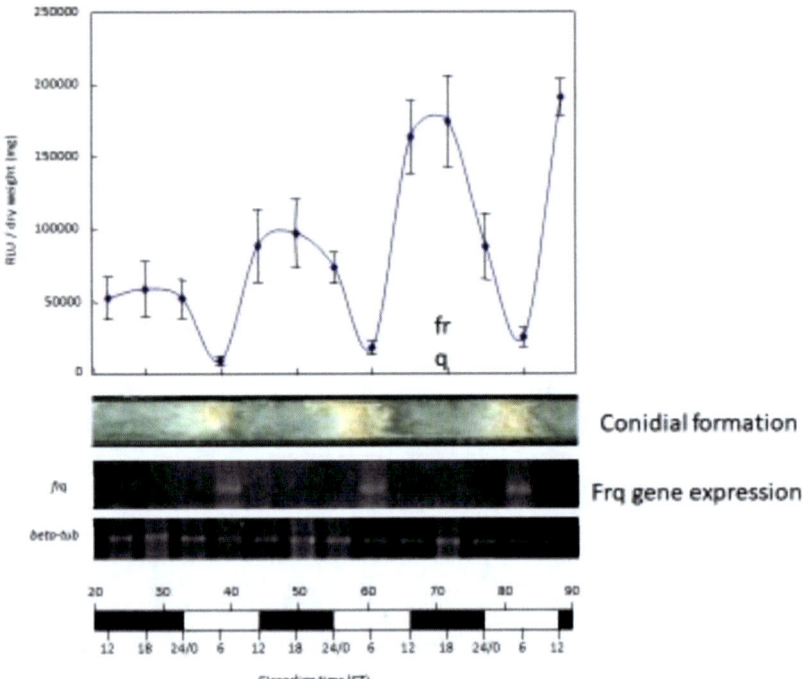

Figure 2.6.2. Circadian oscillation of ROS in the mycelia of *Neurospora crassa*.

Increased [Ca^{2+}]mit will activates three Ca^{2+}-activated dehydrogenases: a pyruvate dehydrogenase, 2-oxoglutarate dehydrogenase, and NAD-dependent isocitrate dehydrogenase. This increases ATP production (Hasunuma, 1991). The energy charges (effective ATP production) in *N. crassa* showed a clear circadian rhythm (Delmer and Brody 1975). Circadian oscillation of the ROS concentration of at the circadian time of late subjective-day (corresponding to late day time) was shown by Yoshida et al. (2011), and the results were presented in Figure 2.6.2.

These results suggest that sunlight triggers singlet oxygen ($^1O_2$) production. Singlet oxygen ($^1O_2$) shows emission in the range 200-500 µm, which can permeate the endoplasmic reticulum and destroy its integrity, releasing Ca^{2+}.

The increase in [Ca^{2+}]cyt triggers an increase in [Ca^{2+}]mt, which serves and finally to increase energy charge (effective ATP production) will also increase. The increase in effective ATP production in the mitochondria is associated with an increased ROS concentration (Yoshida et al. 2011). The precise reaction mechanisms of the ATP production and associated ROS production generation remains unclear, and have not been investigated in detail. The circadian rhythm-based appearance of a high concentration of energy, and resulting high concentration of ROS are challenging clinical problems (Yoshida et al. 2011). The experimental organization and results are presented shown in Figure 2.6.1 and Figure 2.6.2.

The circadian changes in these factors were not examined in all experiments involving humans, and thus additional studies are needed to verify the results. Experiments are needed from the perspective of circadian rhythm, particularly to examine the effects of strong sunlight during the daytime on humans as living model organisms.

The following paper is a high in the quality as a review article published in 2017. However, the singlet oxygen ($^1O_2$) generated by strong sunlight at the daytime on the model system was not considered.

In the review article, Leone et al. (2017) reported that oxidative stress-related gene expression profile correlated with the poor prognosis of cancer patients. Therefore, identification of crucial pathways may assist in selecting novel therapeutic approaches (Prognosis: forecast of the probable course of a disease 予後).

The roles of altered redox status and high ROS levels are controversial with respect to cancer development and progression. Intracellular levels of ROS are elevated in cancer cells, suggesting a role in cancer initiation and progression; in contrast, elevated ROS levels may induce programmed cell death and are associated with cancer suppression. Thus, it is crucial to consider the dual role of ROS, when developing novel therapeutic strategies targeting redox regulatory mechanisms. In this review, the author integrated a publicly available oxidative stress-related gene signature with patient survival data from "The Cancer Genome Atlas database" to derive cancer-type specific oxidative stress-related genes' profiles and identify their potential prognostic roles. Overall, the author detected several genes significantly associated with poor prognosis in the six examined tumor types. Among them, FoxM1 (Forkhead box M1) and (1) thioredoxin reductase1 expression showed the same pattern in four out of six cancers, suggesting their specific critical roles in cancer-related oxidative stress adaptation. Analysis also revealed an enriched cellular network, highlighting specific pathways, in which many genes were strictly correlated. Finally, the author describes novel findings regarding the correlation between oxidative stress and cancer stem cells in order to define the pathways that should be prioritized for drug development. Data regarding the microenvironment-mediated deregulation of ROS are available; however, studies have recently been conducted in this field. In this regard, Chan et al (2017). demonstrated that cancer-associated fibroblast- (CAF-)- derived ROS are able to induce the acquisition of an oxidative CAF-like state in normal fibroblasts. Subsequently, these oxidatively transformed normal fibroblasts promote the development of aggressive tumors via a TGFβ1-mediated Smad3 signaling, suggesting an important relationship between the extracellular redox state and cancer aggressiveness. (1) Thioredoxin reductases (TR, TrxR) are the only known enzymes that to reduce thioredoxin (Trx). The enzyme catalyzes the -S-S- bonds of the protein to –SH + HS-.

Information on peroxidases from Wikipedia
Peroxidases (EC number 1.11.1.x) are a large family of enzymes that typically catalyze a reaction as shown below:

$$ROOR' + 2e^- \text{(electron donor)} + 2H^+ \rightarrow \text{peroxidase} \rightarrow ROH + R'OH$$

For many of these enzymes, the optimal substrate is hydrogen peroxide, while others are more active using organic hydroperoxides such as lipid peroxides as substrates. Peroxidases can contain a heme cofactor in their active sites, or alternately redox-active cysteine or selenocysteine residues. The nature of the electron donor is very dependent on the enzyme structure. For example, horseradish peroxidase can use a variety of organic compounds as electron donors and acceptors. Horseradish peroxidase contains an accessible active site, and many compounds can reach the site of the reaction. On the contrary, for an enzymes with narrow active sites, such as cytochrome C peroxidase, only specific compounds can donate electrons are very specific, due to a very narrow active site.

1) Animal heme-dependent peroxidases
2) Ascorbate peroxidase: (Partly referred in this book)
3) Catalase: **(Referred in this book)**
4) Chloride peroxidase: (Partly referred in this book)
5) Cytochrome C peroxidase
6) Glutathione peroxidase: (Patly referred in this book)
7) Haloperoxidase

8) Hemoprotein
9) Lactoperoxidase
10) Manganese peroxidase
11) Myeloperoxidase (MPO): (Referred in this book)
12) Peroxide
13) Peroxiredoxin
14) Thyroid peroxidase
15) Vanadium bromoperoxidase
16) Sereno-peroxidase

This information is partially based on the description available from Wikipedia.

All of these enzymes bind heme and may bind singlet oxygen ($^1O_2$).

2.7. The Myeloperoxidase (MPO): In Humans Is Encoded by the *MPO* Gene on Chromosome 17 (Q22, Long Arm, Position 22)

MPO is an iron heme protein and homodimer, with a molecular mass of 150-kDa molecular mass. MPO has a Ca^{2+} binding site of 96 Asp residues close to the catalytic site of His 95. MPO catalyzes the following reaction: of,

Chloride (Cl^-) + Hydrogen peroxide (H_2O_2) + H^+ → $HClO$ + H_2O

HClO is (hypochlorous acid), possesses strong activity of bactericidal activity, and is toxic to other pathogens.

In this section, the author describes myeloperoxidase and also the surrounding enzymes, including glutathione peroxidase.

The summary of these phenomena in response of these enzymes to sunlight at daytime, followed by that at nighttime is presented in Figure 2.5.1 and Figure 2.5.2.

Summary of these phenomena in response of these enzymes to sunlight during the daytime, followed by that at nighttime, is presented in Figure 2.6.2.

The following three papers are presented to better understanding of the topic.

Heslop et al. (2010) reported that myeloperoxidase and C-reactive protein have combined utility for long-term prediction of cardiovascular (心臓血管系の) mortality after coronary (冠のような形をした) angiography (血管造影法). Briefly, they found that oxidative stress participates in all stages of cardiovascular disease, from lipoprotein modification to plaque rupture, and biomarkers of oxidative stress predict the development of coronary artery (動脈) disease (CAD). Oxidative stress biomarkers merit investigation for their potential value in long-term cardiovascular risk prediction.

Kutter et al. (2000) reported the consequences (risk versus benefit) of total and subtotal myeloperoxidase deficiency. They examined a group of 100 totally or subtotally myeloperoxidase (MPO)-deficient individuals and compared to a reference population of 118 randomly selected probands. The results suggest a protective effect of the deficiency against cardiovascular damage associated with this deficiency, particularly in probands (particularly a person in the family).

Marrocco et al. (2017) reported a review article regarding the measurement and clinical significance of biomarkers of oxidative stress in humans. Oxidative stress is the result of an imbalance between ROS formation and the availability of enzymatic and nonenzymatic antioxidants. Biomarkers of oxidative stress are relevant for evaluating the disease status and determining the health-enhancing effects of antioxidants. The author describes the major bias of methods used to evaluate oxidative stress in humans. There is a lack of consensus regarding the validation (妥当性), standardization, and reproducibility of methods used to measure the following:

(1) ROS in leukocytes and platelets by flow cytometry,
(2) markers based on ROS-induced modifications of lipids, DNA, and proteins,
(3) enzymatic players in the redox status, and
(4) total antioxidant capacity of human body fluids.

It has been suggested that the bias in each method can be overcome by using indices of oxidative stress that include more than one marker. However, the choice of markers for inclusion in the global index should be determined based on the aim of the study and its design, as well as by the clinical relevance in the selected subjects. In conclusion, the clinical significance of biomarkers of oxidative stress in humans must be determined by critical analysis of the markers to provide an overall index of redox status under specific conditions.

2.8. Use of B-Cell and T-Cell Systems for Controlling Cancerous Cells

The classification of Wikipedia has been explained. Tumor antigens are antigenic substances produced by tumor cells, and trigger an immune response in the host. Tumor antigens are useful as diagnostic tumor markers for identifying tumor cells using diagnostic tests, and are potential candidates for use in cancer therapy. The field of cancer immunology encompasses studies on such topics.

Normal proteins in the body are not antigenic because of self-tolerance, a process in which self-reacting cytotoxic T lymphocytes (CTLs) and autoantibody-producing B lymphocytes are removed centrally from primary lymphatic tissue (BM: bone marrow (骨髄) and peripherally from secondary lymphatic tissue (mostly thymus for T-cells and spleen/lymph nodes for B cells). Thus, any protein that is not exposed to the immune system triggers an immune response. This may include normal proteins that are well sequestered from the immune system, proteins that are normally produced in extremely small quantities, proteins that are normally produced or only in certain stages of development, or mutated proteins whose structures are modified because of mutations.

Tumor antigens are broadly classified into two categories based on their pattern of expression:

a) Tumor-specific antigens (TSA), which are present only on tumor cells and not on any other cell.
b) Tumor-associated antigens (TAA), which are present on some tumor cells and on some normal cells.

This classification, however, is imperfect as many antigens thought to be tumor-specific were found to be expressed on some normal cells as well. The modern classification of tumor antigens is based on their molecular structure and source.

Accordingly, these cells can be classified as follows.

Products of mutated oncogenes and tumor-suppressor genes

1) Products of other mutated genes
2) Overexpressed or aberrantly expressed cellular proteins
3) Tumor antigens produced by oncogenic viruses
4) Oncofetal antigens (proteins that are typically present only during fetal development but are found in adults with certain types of cancer)
5) Altered cell surface glycolipids and glycoproteins
6) Cell type-specific differentiation antigens

Table 2.8.1. Because of their relative abundance, tumor cells are useful for identifying specific tumor types. Tumors have antigens specific for the tumor type, where they are expressed in abundance

Tumor Antigen	Tumor in which it is found	Remarks
Alpha fetoprotein (AFP)	Germ cell tumors Hepatocellular carcinoma	
Carcinoembryonic antigen (CEA)	Bowel caners	Occasional lung or breast cancer
CA-125	Ovarian cancers	Occasional lung or breast cancer
MUC-1, Epithelial tumor antigen (ETA)	Breast cancer	
Tyrosinase	Malignant melanoma	Normally present in minute quantities; highly elevated in melanoma
Melanoma-associated antigen (MAGE)	Malignant melanoma	Normally present in the testis
Abnormal products of ras, p53	Various tumors	

Typical tumor antigens are shown in Table 2.8.1.

Dome tumor antigens are thus used as tumor markers. More importantly, tumor antigens can be used in cancer therapy as tumor antigen vaccines. T lymphocytes are immune system cells that attack and destroy virus-infected cells, tumor cells, and cells from transplanted organs. This occurs because each T cell harbors a highly specific receptor that can bind to an antigen present on the surface of another cell. The T cell receptor binds to a complex formed by a surface protein named MHC (major histocompatibility complex) and small peptide of approximately nine amino-acids, which is located in a groove of the MHC molecule. This peptide can originate from an intracellular protein that remains within the cell. Whereas each T cell recognizes a single antigens, collectively, the T cells show high diversity of receptors targeting a wide variety of antigens. T cells originate in the thymus. A process named as central tolerance eliminates T cells that express a receptor recognizing an antigen present on normal cells in the organism. This enables T cells to eliminate cells with "foreign" or "abnormal" antigens without harming normal cells.

Whether cancer cells express "tumor-specific" antigens that are, absent from normal cells, which can be targeted by the immune system to eliminate the tumor, is highly debated. Evidence has shown that tumor-specific antigens exist and that patients' mount (装置する) spontaneous T cell responses against such antigens. Unfortunately, in many and perhaps most instances, this response is insufficient to prevent cancer progression and metastasis. The purpose of T cell-mediated cancer immunotherapy is to reactivate these responses to a degree that results in tumor destruction without causing harm normal cells.

Fundamentally, we would like to apply this tumor-originated antigen system for eliminating tumors *in vivo*. The vigorously dividing ability of cancerous cells can be suppressed by the administration of several detoxification materials at the cancerous cells, such as

1) Unsaturated fatty acids
2) Nm23-H1 and Nm23-H2 proteins
3) Catalase
4) Cu, Zn-SOD-3
5) Tocopherol: (Vitamin E)
6) Vitamin C
7) Beta-carotene.

However, the amount of doses, and concentrations of administered drugs should be determined from preliminary experiments by using these reagents, cancerous cell lines, appropriate T-cells, and B-cells.

He et al. (2014) reviewed the roles of regulatory B cells in cancer. Regulatory B cells (Bregs), a newly described subset of B cells, were shown to play a suppressive role in the immune system. Bregs can inhibit other immune cells via cytokine secretion and antigen presentation processes, which endow them with definite roles in the pathogenesis of autoimmune diseases and cancers. There are no clear criteria for identifying Bregs, and different markers have been used under varying experimental conditions. Many research reports have described the functions of immune cells such as regulatory T cells (Tregs), dendritic cells (DCs 樹状の), and B cells in autoimmune disorder diseases and cancers. Currently, an increasing numbers of studies has focused on the roles of Bregs and cytokines such as interleukin-10 (IL-10) and transforming growth factor beta (TGF-β), which show increased secretion by Bregs. The aim of this review is to summarize the characteristics of Bregs and their roles in cancer pathogenesis.

REFERENCES

Becuwe, P., Ennen, M., Klotz, R., Barbieux, C. and Grandemange, S. 2014. Manganese superoxide dismutase in breast cancer: from molecular mechanisms of gene regulation to biological and clinical significance. *Free Radic. Biol. Med.* 77:139-151.

Bhattacharya, S. 2015. Reactive oxygen species and cellular defense system. Book. *Free Radicals and Oxidative Stress in Neurodegenerative Disorders,* pp.17-25.

Birben, E., Sahiner, U. M., Sackesen, C., Erzurum, S. and Kalayci, O. 2012. *Oxdative Stress and Antioxidant Defence.* 5(1): 9-19.

Boissan, M., De Wever, O., Lizarraga, F., Wendum, D., Poincloux, R., Chignard, N., Desbois-Mouthon, C., Dufour, S., Nawrocki-Reby, B., Birembaut, P., Bracke, M., Chavrier, P., Gespach, C. and Lacombe, M. L. 2010. Implication of metastasis suppressor NM23-H1 in maintaining adherens junctions and limiting the invasive potential of human cancer cells. *Cancer Res.* 70 (19): 7710-7722.

Bosnar, M. H., Bago, R. and Cetkovic, H. 2009. Subcellular localization of Nm23/NDPK A and B isoforms: a reflection of their biological function? *Mol. Cell. Biochem.* 329(1-2): 63-71.

Boso, G., Ke, D., Korzh, B., Bouilloux, J., Lange, N. and Zbinden, H. 2016. Time-resolved singlet-oxygen luminescence detection with an efficient and practical semiconductor single-photon detector. *Biomed. Opt. Exp.* 7(1): 211-224.

Buxton, I. L. O. and Nordmeier, S. 2015. Rethinking NM23: An extracellular role for NDPKinase in breast cancer. *Integrative Cancer Sci. and Therap.* 2 (3): 153-157.

Chan, J. S. K., Tan, M, J., Sng, M. K., Teo, Z., Phua, T., Choo, C. C., Ll, L., Zhu, P. and Tan, N. S. 2017. Cancer-associated fibroblasts enact field cancerization by promoting extratumoral oxidative stress. Cell Death Dis. 8 (1): e2562

Deaton, A. M. and Bird, A. 2011. CpG islands and the regulation of transcription. *Genes and Dev.* 25: 1010-1022.

Delmer, D. P. and Brody, S. 1975. Circadian rhythms in *Neurospora crassa*: oscillation in the level of an adenine nucleotide. *J. Bacteriol.* 121(2): 548-553.

Ding, Z.-C. and Zhou, G. 2012. Review Article: Cytotoxic chemotherapy and CD4+ effector T cells: an emerging alliance for durable antitumor effects. *Clinical and Developmental Immunology.* vol. 20122012:, Article ID 890178, 12 pages.

Forsberg, L., Lyrenas, L., Morgenstern, R. and Faire, U. 2001. A common functional C-T substitution polymorphism in the promoter region of the human catalase gene influences transcription factor binding, reporter gene transcription and is correlated to blood catalase levels. *Free Rad. Biol. and Med.* 30(5): 500-505.

Giraud, M.-F., Georgescauld, F., Lascu, I. and Dautan, A. 2006. Crystal structure of S120G mutant and wild type of human nucleoside diphosphate kinase A in complex with ADP. *J. Bioener. and Biomemb.* 38. 261.

Glorieux, C., Sandoval, J. M., Dejeans, N., Nonckreman, S., Bahloula, K., Poirel, H. A. and Calderon, P. B. 2018. Evaluation of potential mechanisms controlling the catalase expression in breast cancer cells. *Oxid. Med. Cell Longev.* 2018: 5351967.

Goth, L., Nagy, T. and Kaplar, M. 2015. Acatalasemia and type 2 diabetes mellitus. *Orv. Hetil.* 156(10): 393-398.

Goth, L., Rass, P. and Pay, A. 2004. Catalase enzyme mutations and their association with diseases. *Mol. Diagn.* 8(3): 141-149.

Gu, Z., Suburu, J., Chen, H. and Chen, Y. Q. 2013. Mechanism of omega-3 polyunsaturated fatty acids in prostate cancer prevention. *Biomed. Res. Int.* 2013: 824563.

Hackenberg, T., Juul, T., Auzina, A., Guizdz, S., Malolepszy, A., Van Der Kelen, K., Dam, S., Bressendorff, S., Lorenzen, A., Roepstorff, P., Nielsen, K. L., Jorgensen, J-E., Hofius, D., Breusegen, F. A., Petersen, M. and Andersen, S. U. 2013. Catalase and No Catalase Activity 1 promote autophagy-dependent cell death in Arabidopsis. *The Plant Cell,* 27: 1-11.

Hasunuma, K. 2017. Detoxification of singlet oxygen: Raising up crop yield and the clinical application, *Advances in Medicine and Biology,* Chapter 5, Vol. 121, pp. 115-132. Ed; Leon V. Berhardt, Nova Science Publisher, Co., Ltd. New York.

Hasunuma, K. 1991. Molecular mechanism of light signal perception in plants and fungi. *Trends in Photochem. Photobiol.* 1: 311-319.

Hasunuma, K. and Shinohara, Y. 1987. Circadian rhythm of *Neurospora crassa* (2) *Iden* (genetics) 41 (2): 48-57. (written in Japanese)

He, Y., Qian, H., Liu, Y., Duan, L., Li, Y. and Shi. G. 2014. Review Article: The roles of regulatory B cells in cancer. *J. Immun. Res.* vol. 2014:, Article ID 215471, 7 pages.

Heslop, C. L., Frohlich, J. J. and Hill, J. S. 2010. Myeloperoxidase and C-reactive protein have combined utility for long-term prediction of cardiovascular mortality after coronary angiography. *J. Am. Coll. Cardiol.* 55(11): 1102-1109.

Hsu, T., Steeg, P. S., Zollo, M. and Wieland, T. 2015. Progress on Nme (NDP kinase/Nm23/*Awd*) gene family-related functions derived from animal model systems: studies on development, cardiovascular disease, and cancer metastasis exemplified. *Naunyn-Schmiedeberg's Arch Phamacol.* 388: 109-117.

Hwang, G. B., Park, I. C., Park, M. J., Moon, N. M., Choi, D. W., Hong, W. S., Lee, S. H. and Hong, S. I. 1997. Role of the nm23-H1 gene in the metastasis of gastric cancer. *J. Korean Med. Sci.* 12(6): 514-518.

Iguchi, T. and Takasugi, N. 1986. Polyovular follicles in the ovary of immature mice exposed prenatally to diethylstilbestrole. *Anat. Embryol.* 175: 53–55.

Ito, Y., Kawamorita, M., Yamabe, T., Kiyono, T. and Miyamoto, K. 2007. Chemically fixed nurse cells for culturing murine or primate embryonic stem cells. *J. Biosci. Bioengineering.* 103 (2): 113-121.

Jank. S. J., Shin, W. J., Lee, J. E. and Do, J. T. 2017. CpG and non-CpG methylation in epigenetic gene regulation and brain function. *Genes* (Basel), vol. 8, no. (6)8: 148.

Kamogashira, T., Fujimoto, C. and Yamasoba, T. 2015. Reactive oxygen species, apoptosis, and mitochondrial dysfunction in hearing loss. *Biomed. Res. Int.* 2015: 617207.

Khan, F. H., Pandian, V., Ramraj, S. K., Aravindan, S., Natarajan, M., Azadi, S., Herman, T. S. and Aravindan, N. 2015. RD3 loss dictates high-risk aggressive neuroblastoma and poor clinical outcomes. *Oncotarget.* 6(34): 36522-36534.

Khan. I. and Steeg, P. S. 2017. Tumor Biology, Abstract 1047: Role of endocytosis in NM23 mediated motility suppression. *Cancer Res.* 77 (13 supplement: Proceedings)

Kirkman, H. N., Galiano, S. and Gaetani, G. F. 1987. The function of catalase-bound NADPH. *J. Biol. Chem.,* 262(2): 660-666.

Kosa, Z., Fejes, Z., Nagy, T., Csordas, M., Simics, E., Remenyik, E. and Goth, L.2012. Catalase -262C>T polymorphysms in Hungarian vitiligo patients and in controls: further acatalasemia mutations in

Hungary. *Mol. Biol. Rep.* 39(4): 4787-4795. (Vitiligo: white spot in skin)

Kowluru, A., Tannous, M. and Chen, H. Q. 2002. Localization and characterization of the mitochondrial isoform of the nucleoside diphosphate kinase in the pancreatic beta cell: evidence for its complexation with mitochondrial succinyl-CoA synthetase. *Arch. Biochem. Biophys.* 398(2): 160-169.

Kutter, D., Devaquet, P., Vanderstocken, G., Paulus, J. M., Marchal, V. and Gothot, A. 2000. Consequences of total and subtotal myeloperoxidase deficiency: risk or benefit? *Acta Haematol.* 104(1): 10-15.

Krueger, K., Shen, J., Maier, A., Tepel, M. and Sholze, A. 2016. Lower Superoxide Dismutase 2 (SOD2) protein content in mononuclear cells is associated with better survival in patients with hemodialysis therapy. *Dxid. Med. Cell. Longev.* PMC5007362.

Lahiri, B. M., Rogers, J. T. and Ge, Y-W. 2013. Puf, an antimetastatic and developmental signaling protein, interacts with the Alzheimer's amyloid-beta precursor protein via a tissue-specific proximal regulatory element (PRE). *BMC Genomics* 14: 68.

Leone, A., Roca, M. S., Ciardiello, C., Costantini, S. and Budillon, A. 2017. Oxidative stress gene expression profile correlates with cancer patient poor prognosis: identification of crucial pathways might select novel therapeutic approaches. *Oxid. Med. Cell Longev.* 2017. 2597581.

Liang, Q., Wei, D., Chung, B., Brulois, K. F., Guo, C., Dong, S., Gao, S. J. Feng, P., Liang, C. and Jung, J. U. 2018 J. Virol. Novel role of vBcl2 in the viron assembly of Kaposi's sarcoma-associated herpesvirus. *J. Virol.* 92(4). Pii: e00914-e00917.

Lin, J., Cook, N. R., Albert, C., Zaharris, E., Gaziano, J. M., Denburgh, M. V., Buring, J. E. and Manson. J.-A. E. 2009. Vitamins C and E and beta carotene supplementation and cancer risk: a randomized controlled trial. *J. Natl. Cancer Inst.* 101(1): 14–23.

Liu, L., Zhou, Q., Sun, Z., Qin, Y., Shi, Y. and Sun, Z. 2000. Mutational analysis of nm23-H1 gene in human lung cancer by polymerase chain reaction-single strand conformation polymorphism. *Zhongguo Fei Ai Za Zhi* 3(3): 201-204.

Loep, L. A., Loeb, K. R. and Anderson, J. P. 2003. Multple mutations and cancer. *Proc. Natl. Acad. Sci. USA*. 100(3): 776-781.

Manne, N. D. P. K., Arvapalli, R., Nepal, N., Shokuhfar, T., Rice, K. M., Asano, S. and Blough, E. R. 2015. Cerium oxide nanoparticles attenuate acute kidney injury induced by intra-abdominal infection in Sprague–Dawley rats. *J. Nanobiotech.* 13:75.

Marrocco, I., Altieri, F. and Peluso. I. 2017. Review Article. Measurement and clinical significance of biomarkers of oxidative stress in humans. *Oxida. Med. Cell. Longe.* Article ID 6501046, 32 pages.

Mates, J. M., Perez-Gemez, C., Munez de Castro, I., Asenjo, M. and Marquez, J. 2002. Review. Glutamine and its relationship with intracellular redox status, oxidative stress and cell proliferation/ death. *The Intern. J. Biochem. & Cell Biol.* 34: 439-458.

Mehta, A. and Orchard, S. 2009. Nucleoside diphosphate kinase (NDPK, NM23, *AWD*): recent regulatory advances in endocytosis, metastasis, psoriasis, insulin release, fetal erythroid lineage and heart failure; translational medicine exemplified. *Mol. Cell. Biochem.* 329 (1-2): 3-15.

Mishra, S., Jakkara, K., Srinivasan, R., Arumugan, M., Ranjeri, R., Gupta, P., Rajeswari, H. and Ajitkumar, P. 2015. NDK interacts with FtsZ and converts GDP to GTP to trigger FtsZ. Polymerization-A novel role for NDK. *PLoS One* 10(12): e0143677.

Montero, J. and Letai, A. 2018. Why do BCL-2 inhibitors work and where should we use in the clinic? *Cell Death Differ.* 25(1): 56-64.

Muller, W., Schneiders, A., Hommel, G., and Gabbert, H. E. 1998. Expression of nm23 in gastric carcinoma. Association with tumor progression and poor prognosis. *Cancer*, 83(12): 2481-2487.

Nagy, T., Paszti, E., Kaplar, M., Bhattoa, H. P. and Goth, L. 2015. Further acatalasemia mutations in human patients from Hungary with diabetes and microcytic anemia. *Mutat. Res.* 772(Feb): 10-14.

Nigg, E. A. and Raff J. W. 2009. Centrioles, centrosomes, and cilia in health and disease. *Cell.* 139(4): 663-678.

Pedelsen, W. A. and Mattson, M. P. 1999. No benefit of dietary restriction on disease onset or progression in amyotrophic sclerosis Cu/Zn-superoxide dismutase mutant mice. *Brain Res.* 833(1): 117-120.

Postel, E. H. and Ferrone, C. A. 1994. Nucleoside diphosphate kinase enzyme activity of NM23-H2/PuF is not required for its DNA binding and in vitro transcriptional functions. *J. Biol. Chem.* 269(12): 8627-8630.

Putnam, C. D., Arvai, A. S., Bourne, Y. and Tainer, J. A. 2000. Active and inhibited human catalase structures: ligand and NADPH binding and catalytic mechanism. *J. Mol. Biol.* 296(1): 295-309.

Qui. L., Tan, X., Lin, J., Liu, R. Y., Chen, S., Geng, R., Wu, J. and Huang, W. 2017. CDC27 induces metastasis and invasion in colorectal cancer via the promotion of epithelial-to-messenchymal transition. *J. Cancer* 8(13): 2626-2635.

Rodgers, M. A., Bowman, J. W., Liang, Q. and Jung, J. U. 2013. Regulation where autophagy intersects the inflammasome. *Antioxid. Redox Signal.* 20(3): 495-506.

Roymans, D., Willems, R., Van Blockstaele, D. R. and Sleger, H. 2002. Nucleoside diphosphate kinase (NDPK/NM23) and the waltz with multiple partners: possible consequences in tumor metastasis. *Clin. Exp. Metastasis.* 19(6): 465-476.

Roymans, D., Willems, R., Vissenberg, K., De Jonghe, C., Grobben, B., Claes, P., Lascu, I., Van Bockstaele. D., Verbelen, J. P., Van Broeckhoven, C. and Slegers, H. 2000. Nucleoside diphosphate kinase beta, (Nm23-R1/NDPKbeta) is associated with intermediate filaments and becomes upregulated upon cAMP-induced differentiation of rat C6 glioma. *Exp. Cell. Res.* 261(1): 127-138.

Sakaki, T., Saito, K., Kawaguchi, A., Kondo, N. and Yamada, M. 1990. Conversion of monogalactosyl diacyldiacylglycerols to triacylglycerols in ozone-fumigated Spinach leaves. *Plant Physiology* 94: 766-772.

Schneider-Stock, R., Fakhoury, I. H., Zaki, A. M., El-Baba, C. O. and Gali-Mutasib, H. U. 2014. Thymoquinone: fifty years of success in the battle against cancer models. *Drug Discovery Today.* 19(1): 16-30.

Song, F., Smith, J. F., Kimura, M. T., Morrow, A. D., Matsuyama, T., Nagase, H. and Held, A. A. 2004. Association of tissue-specific differentially methylated regions (TDM) with differential gene expression. *Proc. Natl. Acad. Sci,* USA. 102(9): 3336-3341.

Tan, D.-X., Manchester, L. C., Reiter, R. J., Qi, W.-B., Karbownik, M. and Calvo, J. R. 2000. Significance of melatonin in antioxidative defence system: reactions and products. *Biol. Signals Receipt.* 9: 137-159.

Tong, L. Y., Yung, Y. Y. and Wong, H. 2015. Metastasis suppressors Nm23H1 and Nm23H2 differently regulate neoplastic transformation and tumorigenesis. *Cancer Res.* 361(2): 207-217.

Trachootham, D., Alexandre, J. and Huang, J. 2009. Review. Targetting cancer cells by ROS-mediated mechanism: a radical therapeutic approach? Nature Nat. Reviews Rev. *Drug Discovery.* Vol. 8: 579-591.

Wang, L., Patel, U., Ghosh, L., Chen, H. C. and Banerjee, S. 1993. Mutation in the nm23 gene is associated with metastasis in colorectal cancer. *Cancer Res.* 53(4): 717-720.

Woodruff, J. B., Ferreira Gomes, B., Widlund, P. O., Mahamid, J., Honigmann, A. and Hyman, A. A. 2017. The centrosome is a selective condensate that nucleates microtubules by concentrating tubulin. *Cell* 169 (6): 1066-1077.

Xiong, Z. and Laird, P. W. 1997. COBRA: a sensitive and quantitative DNA methylation assay. *Nucleic Acids Res.,* 25:(12) 2532 – 2534.

Yoshida, Y., Ogura, Y. and Hasunuma, K. 2006. Interaction of nucleoside diphosphate kinase and catalases for stress and light responses in *Neurospora crassa. FEBS Lett.,* 580: 3282-3286.

Yoshida, Y., Iigusa, H., Wang, N. and Hasunuma, K. 2011. Cross-talk between the cellular redox state and the circadian system in Neurospora. *PLoS ONE,* vol. 6, (12): no. e28227; 1-11.

Zhong, H. H. and McClung, C. R. 1996. The circadian clock gates expression of two Arabidopsis catalase genes to distinct and opposite circadian phases. *Mol. Genet. Genomics,* 251(2): 196-203.

CONCLUDING REMARKS

Compared to the results obtained for *N. crassa*, studies of the existing levels of human cancerous cells are limited. The author is a geneticist who graduated with a Japanese Doctorate of Science degree from "The University of Tokyo, in Japan," where he initially intended to analyze and understand photosynthesis, and studied the quantum physics of light at the University. In the case of *N. crassa*, the effects attributed to the experimental conditions of light illumination or exposure to darkness were thoroughly analyzed. In humans, however, experimental conditions cannot be pre-determined. Individuals are regulated by a specific circadian rhythm, which varies based on darkness during the nighttime and strong sunlight during the daytime because of the rotation of the earth. Patients are also exposed to specific living conditions and visit hospitals when they feel unwell: however, they may also be asymptomatic. This situation indicates body-calling diseases; in some cases, this is the first moment of detection of cancerous cells in the body. Without evaluating the situations of the patients, a medical doctor observes the patients critically and determines the diagnoses before diagnosing the disease. The physician makes his diagnosis and shares the information. After providing patients with information, the doctor prescribes medicines, and observes the results of patients after a periodic clinical evaluation of each patient and gives a prognosis of the disease.

1) All patients and healthy individuals should be treated based on the changes of enzymes as per the sunlight received during the day and night cycle, and the data collected after considering the circadian rhythm, including the ages of patients and healthy controls. This system should be established in all hospitals to obtain reliable data.
2) Data collection related to the circadian rhythm should be collected from both patients and healthy individuals, and the data should be compared to that of healthy persons using appropriate statistical methods. The final significance of the differences in results should be determined.
3) All parts of the body can sense light. Temperatures, including both ambient and body temperatures, should be recorded, as singlet oxygen evolution is affected by the environmental temperatures.
4) Final data should be strictly compared statistically and their significance in statistics should be determined.
5) We propose that the DNA sequences of newborns should be checked with approximately 100 species related to humans, mainly with respect to quantum biology and molecular biology, and the data should be used to generate health opinions for future health checkup determinations.

ABOUT THE AUTHOR

Kohji Hasunuma
Professor Emeritus
Yokohama City University
Chairman
Institute of High Yielding Crop Co. Ltd.
Machida, Tokyo Japan
kohji.hasunuma@gmail.com

INDEX

A

abnormal wing disc formation (*AWD*), x, 74
acid, 49, 63
activity level, 39
aggressiveness, 51, 62
amyotrophic lateral sclerosis, 42, 43, 48
angiography, 64, 71
animal science, xi
antigen, 67, 68, 69
antioxidant, 43, 48, 56, 65
Arabidopsis thaliana, 3, 12
ATP, 1, 5, 23, 45, 58, 60
autoimmune diseases, 69

B

biological markers, 45
biomarkers, 46, 64, 65, 74
bone marrow, 65
brain, 44, 72
breast cancer, 45, 56, 69, 70, 71

C

cancer, xv, xvi, 45, 51, 52, 53, 56, 61, 65, 66, 67, 68, 69, 70, 71, 72, 73, 74, 76
cancer cells, 51, 56, 61, 68, 70, 76
cancer progression, 68
cancer stem cells, 61
cancer therapy, 65, 67
cancerous cells, x, xv, xvi, 28, 35, 47, 49, 50, 52, 53, 54, 68, 79
cardiovascular disease, 64, 72
cardiovascular risk, 64
carotene, xvi, 68, 73
carotenoids, 20, 21, 22, 23
cell surface, 66
centriole, 42
centrosome, 41, 76
chemical, 44
chloroplast thylakoids, ix
chromosome, 38, 43, 44, 54, 56
chronic kidney disease (CKD), 46
cilia, 40, 41, 42, 75
cilium, 40
circadian rhythms, x, xiv, 31, 70
classification, 65, 66

clinical application, 29, 71
clinical problems, 60
compounds, xiii, 43, 62
CpG island-controlled genes, x
CpG island-independent genes, x
CpG islands, x, xi, xiv, xv, xvi, 21, 27, 29, 36, 37, 38, 43, 45, 52, 53, 70

D

database, 61
defence, 76
deficiency, 64, 73
dendritic cell, 69
deregulation, 41, 61
derivatives, x, xi, xv, 56
desorption, 44
destruction, 41, 68
detection, 2, 3, 44, 70, 79
detoxification, x, xv, xvi, 18, 29, 39, 45, 50, 52, 54, 55, 68, 71
diseases, xiv, 39, 42, 45, 52, 54, 56, 69, 71, 79
docosahexaenoic acid, 52
doctors, 42
Drosophila melanogaster, x
drugs, 56, 68
dwarfism, 42

E

eicosapentaenoic acid, 52
electrons, xiii, 36, 38, 44, 54, 62
electrophoresis, 2, 5, 25, 44, 47
embryonic stem cells, 72
emission, 20, 39, 41, 60
encoding, 2, 15, 27, 35, 38, 43, 47, 50, 51, 54, 56
energy, ix, xiii, xiv, 2, 60
environment, xvi, 30, 43
environmental change, 27

enzyme, xiv, 2, 6, 11, 22, 23, 24, 25, 42, 43, 48, 51, 62, 71, 75
epithelial cells, 56
ethanol, 59
eukaryotic, 41
evidence, 73
evolution, x, 56, 80
excitation, ix, xiii, xiv, 45
experimental condition, 69, 79
exposure, 1, 16, 22, 23, 32, 36, 37, 38, 42, 48, 49, 53, 57, 79

F

FAD (flavin adenine dinucleotide), x, xi, xiii, xiv, xv, 5, 12, 37, 38, 45, 56
fatty acids, ix, xiii, xvi, 47, 49, 52, 58, 68
fetal development, 66
FMN (flavin mononucleotide), x
formation, x, 3, 9, 19, 41, 48, 64
fungi, 29, 30, 71

G

gel, 2, 3, 5, 12, 13, 25
gene expression, 15, 38, 43, 45, 46, 56, 61, 73, 76
gene regulation, xv, 46, 56, 69, 72
genes, x, xv, 1, 2, 21, 27, 29, 35, 37, 38, 43, 52, 54, 61, 66, 77
genome, x, xv, 41, 43, 52
gland, 46
growth, 26, 27, 28, 50
growth mechanism, 50

H

haploid, x, xv, 52
harbors, 54, 67
healing, 50, 57

health, 52, 64, 75, 80
heme, x, xi, xiii, xiv, xv, 3, 54, 56, 62, 63
heme groups, x, xi, xiv
hemodialysis, 46, 73
historical character, 5, 6
Homo sapiens, x, 35
homopolymers, 13, 15
human, x, xv, xvi, 8, 27, 29, 48, 52, 54, 65, 70, 73, 74, 75, 79
hydrogen, 18, 26, 31, 39, 44, 46, 55, 62
hydrogen peroxide, 18, 26, 31, 39, 44, 46, 55, 62
hydroperoxides, 62
hydroxyl, 44
hypothesis, 44, 50

I

identification, 40, 44, 61, 73
illumination, xi, 1, 5, 11, 14, 15, 22, 23, 24, 27, 36, 45, 79
immune system, 66, 67, 68, 69
immunoprecipitation, 57
individuals, 17, 38, 64, 79, 80
induction, 15, 16, 17, 20, 21, 22
inflammasome, 75
ionization, 44
islands, x, xi, xiv, xv, xvi, 21, 27, 29, 36, 37, 38, 43, 45, 52, 53, 70

K

karyotype, 56
kidney, 74
kinase activity, 50

L

lateral sclerosis, 42, 48
leukemia, 57

leukocytes, 65
life cycle, 5
ligand, 75
light, 5, xi, 1, 2, 3, 4, 5, 6, 8, 9, 11, 12, 14, 15, 16, 19, 21, 22, 23, 24, 26, 27, 29, 30, 31, 32, 33, 36, 71, 77, 79, 80
lipid peroxides, 62
living conditions, 79
localization, 9, 10, 11, 32, 36, 70
lymph node, 66
lymphocytes, 65

M

major histocompatibility complex, 67
malondialdehyde (MDA), x
manipulation, 48
mass, 13, 44, 63
materials, 41, 68
melatonin, 76
metabolic syndrome, 52
metastasis, xvi, 35, 68, 70, 72, 74, 75, 76
methylation, x, xi, xiv, xv, xvi, 21, 29, 36, 37, 38, 42, 43, 45, 53, 56, 72, 76
mitochondria, 13, 23, 39, 40, 43, 60
mitochondrial envelope, ix
model system, 50, 60, 72
modifications, 42, 47, 57, 65
molecular biology, 5, x, 80
morphogenesis, 9, 20, 25, 43
mortality, 46, 50, 64, 71
motor neuron disease, 42
mRNA, 22, 23, 24, 25, 42, 43, 50, 57
mutant, xiv, 1, 9, 14, 15, 16, 17, 18, 24, 25, 26, 27, 28, 29, 30, 32, 48, 70, 75
mutations, 18, 43, 48, 66, 71, 72, 74

N

neuroblastoma, 38, 72

Neurospora crassa, 7, x, xiv, 1, 29, 30, 31, 32, 33, 35, 58, 59, 70, 71, 77
nuclear membrane, ix, 47
nuclei, 12, 21, 27, 36, 38, 42, 47, 49, 52
Nucleoside diphosphate kinase (NDPK), x
nucleus, xi, 12, 36, 38, 41, 43, 45

O

organic compounds, 62
organism, 20, 68
oscillation, xiv, 59, 60, 70
oxidation, xiv
oxidative stress, 16, 17, 18, 19, 44, 48, 57, 61, 64, 65, 74
oxide nanoparticles, 74
oxygen, ix, xiii, xiv, xv, 3, 4, 18, 21, 27, 29, 32, 36, 37, 39, 41, 42, 46, 54, 55, 56, 58, 60, 63, 69, 70, 71, 72, 80
ozone, 49, 76
ozone-resistant, 49

P

pathways, 43, 46, 61, 73
phenotype, 9, 20, 30, 48
phosphorylation, xiv, 1, 5, 6, 7, 13, 16, 29, 32, 57
photo-activated chlorophyll, ix
photolysis, ix, xiii, xiv
photosensitizers, x, xi, xiii, xiv, xv, 12, 36, 37, 38, 45, 56, 58
photosynthesis, 5, xi, 79
plasma membrane, ix, xi, xiii, 11, 12, 20, 29, 36, 38, 47
platelets, 65
point mutation, xiv, 9, 24, 32, 43
polymerase chain reaction, 47, 74
polyunsaturated fatty acids, 52, 71
porphyrin, xi, xiii, xv
precipitation, 14, 15

prevention, 71
prognosis, 61, 73, 74, 79
proliferation, x, xv, 44, 46, 50, 52, 56, 74
promoter, 42, 50, 70
protein-protein interactions, 13
proteins, xv, xvi, 1, 2, 3, 10, 11, 12, 13, 15, 29, 35, 36, 40, 41, 57, 65, 66, 68
psoriasis, 74

Q

quantum physics, xi, 79

R

reactive oxygen species (ROS), x, xiv, 31, 41, 44
response, 5, 1, 4, 9, 20, 32, 44, 52, 53, 64, 68
reticulum, xiii, 58, 60
rhythm, x, xiv, 4, 32, 58, 71
riboflavin, x, xi, xiii, xiv, xv, 4, 5, 12, 29, 37, 38, 45, 56

S

signal transduction, 30, 31, 32, 40, 50
signaling pathway, 57
singlet oxygen ($^1O_2$), ix, xiii, xiv, xv, 3, 18, 27, 36, 41, 42, 54, 55, 58, 60, 63
sodium dodecyl sulfate (SDS), 2
species, x, xiv, 15, 31, 32, 41, 44, 69, 72, 80
stress, 16, 17, 18, 19, 20, 32, 33, 52, 61, 64, 65, 73, 77
structure, xi, 41, 43, 62, 70
suppression, 31, 35, 61, 72
survival, 46, 47, 50, 61, 73
synthesis, 4, 20, 21, 23, 31

T

T cell, 67, 68, 69, 70
T lymphocytes, 65, 67
tetrapyrrole, xi, xiii, xiv
transcription, 16, 18, 37, 38, 42, 43, 47, 52, 53, 70
transcription factors, 38, 42
transforming growth factor, 69
triggers, 60, 66
triplet chlorophyll, ix, xiv
triplet oxygen ($^3O_2$), ix, xiii, xiv, 39, 56
tubulin structures, xi, 48
tumor, 41, 45, 50, 61, 65, 66, 67, 68, 74, 75
tumor cells, 46, 50, 65, 66, 67
type 2 diabetes, 71

U

unsaturated fatty acids, ix, xiii, xvi, 47, 49, 58

V

viruses, 66
vitamin E, xvi, 49
vitamin K, 56
vitiligo, 72

W

Western blot, 10, 11, 12, 46
wild type, 14, 20, 70
worldwide, 45

Z

zinc, 43

Cancer and Stem Cells

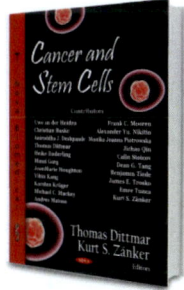

EDITORS: Thomas Dittmar and Kurt S. Zanker (Inst. of Immunology, Witten/Herdecke University, Germany)

SERIES: Cancer Etiology, Diagnosis and Treatments

BOOK DESCRIPTION: The purpose of this book is to summarize the latest findings about the role of stem cells in cancer.

HARDCOVER ISBN: 978-1-60456-478-5
RETAIL PRICE: $150

The Functional and Translational Immunology of Regulatory T Cells (Tregs), the Anti-Tumor T Cell Response, and Cancer

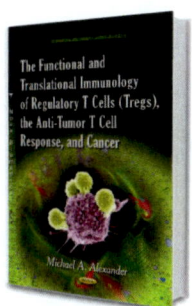

AUTHOR: Michael A. Alexander (Widener University, One University Place, Chester, PA, USA)

SERIES: Immunology and Immune System Disorders

BOOK DESCRIPTION: This book examines the function and related translational pathways of Tregs, anti-tumor T cells, and cancer cells. It relates that information to the treatment of cancer by examining human clinical trials of new immune cell-based treatments (immunotherapy).

HARDCOVER ISBN: 978-1-62808-716-1
RETAIL PRICE: $185

Myeloid Cells: Biology & Regulation, Role in Cancer Progression and Potential Implications for Therapy

Editor: Spencer A. Douglas

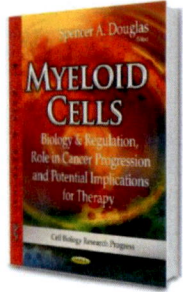

Series: Cell Biology Research Progress

Book Description: In this book the authors present current research in the study of the biology and regulation, role in cancer progression and potential implications for therapy of myeloid cells.

Hardcover ISBN: 978-1-62948-046-6
Retail Price: $110

Therapeutic Potential of Differentiation in Cancer and Normal Stem Cells

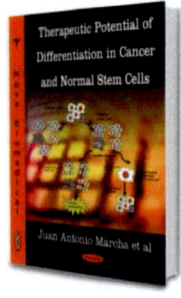

Authors: Juan Antonio Marchal, Houria Boulaiz, Macarena Peran, et al. (University of Granada, Granada, Spain)

Book Description: This new model has important implications for the study and treatment of cancer.

Softcover ISBN: 978-1-60692-917-9
Retail Price: $59